Who Needs Headaches?

Cass Igram, D.O.

Literary Visions Publishing, Inc.
Cedar Rapids, Iowa

ISBN Number 0-911119-32-9

Published by
Literary Visions Publishing

Printed By
Cedar Graphics, Inc.
P.O. Box 1451
Cedar Rapids, IA 52406-1451

For ordering information call:
319-366-5335

DEDICATION

For those who are suffering and wish to suffer no longer.

This book contains information, advice and observations related to the study of migraines and other headaches. This book is not intended as a substitute for medical diagnosis or treatment. The reader who has a serious disease should consult a physician before initiating any change in his/her treatment or before beginning any new treatment.

TABLE OF CONTENTS

INTRODUCTION

CHAPTER 1: What Started All This Pain?

CHAPTER 2: Many Kinds, Many Causes
- Heavy Metals 8
- Drugs and Other Chemicals 9
- Stress, Blood Sugar and Migraine 10
- Intestinal Reflexes 11

CHAPTER 3: Making the Diagnosis
- How to Make a Diagnosis 15
  — Types of Tests

CHAPTER 4: Allergies: The Number One Cause
- The Migraine Personality: Does It Really Exist? 19
- The Allergy-Migraine Connection: A Review of Scientific
  Literature 20
- The Food Intolerance Test: A Simple Method for
  Determining Migraine-Provoking Foods 23
- How Food Allergy Reactions Occur: The Immune
  Connection 25
- Secretory IgA Is the First Line of Defense 27
- The Leaky Gut Syndrome: A Result of Secretory IgA
  Deficiency? 29
- Food Additives: A Major Cause of Allergic Migraines 33
- Sulfites: Culprit Number One 34
- MSG: Culprit Number Two 36
- Food Dyes: Culprit Number Three 39
- Food Additives and the Migraine Patient 41
- Real Food: The Major Cause of Migraines 42
- Mechanisms of Food Allergy: Migraine Reactions 43
- Can Food Allergies Short-Circuit the Brain? 45
- Do Children Have Migraines? 46
- White and Dangerous: Are Artificial Sweeteners
  Headache Promoters? 49
- Your Fillings: Can You Be Allergic to Them? 50
- Food Allergies and Migraine: Selected Case Histories 53

CHAPTER 5: Hormonal Disorders: The Number Two Cause

CHAPTER 6: Structural Therapies
- Manipulation: A Science or An Art? 81
  — Why OMT/CMT works
  — Neck injuries
  — The anatomy of the neck
  — Mid to upper back
  — The lower back
  — The tailbone
- Trigger Point Injections 87
  — How to treat trigger points
  — The technique
  — What is injected?
  — How much is injected?
  — Who can do it?
  — Why trigger point therapy works
  — How do painful triggers arise?

CHAPTER 7: Nutrients and Migraines
- Herbs 93
- Minerals 95
- Calcium: The Nerve Tonic Material 97
- Magnesium: Migraine Blocking Agent 100
- Chromium: Blood Sugar Regulating Mineral 101
- Vitamins 102
  — Pantothenic Acid: Vitamin Powerhouse
  — Vitamin B-6: Nature's Diuretic
  — Vitamin C: The Natural Antihistamine
  — Vitamin E: Blood Flow Performer
- Amino Acids 105
- Tyrosine Prevents Hormone and Neurotransmitter
  Deficiency 106
- Enzymes 107
- Enzymes, Allergy and Migraine 108
- Fish Oils: Supplement #1 for Migraines 109
- GLA: The Other Anti-Migraine Fatty Acid 112

CHAPTER 8: Conclusion

INTRODUCTION

Migraine headaches are one of the major plagues of modern civilization. Millions of people all over the world are afflicted with this dreaded illness. However, migraines as well as most other types of headaches are more common in the USA than anywhere in the world.

Though migraine headaches are among the most common of the ailments afflicting modern man, they are not a new disease. Rather, they have existed for thousands of years. The ancient Egyptians and Greeks experienced them. Back then, no one really knew the cause. Yet, the ancients did ponder over the possibility that food reactions were partly to blame. Just what caused the pain of migraine remained an enigma over the remaining centuries until 1913 when two Frenchmen, Doctors Lesne and Richet, proposed that *food allergy* was the likely culprit.

Unfortunately, few took note of their observation. To this day the cause of migraines continues to remain unknown to most medical researchers and practitioners.

In the past, treatments for migraine headaches have been crude and ineffective. Everything from surgery to herbs and poultices have been tried to no avail. The reason these treatments failed was that they neglected to address the cause. The sufferers of old found little or no relief for their migraines. They didn't even have Tylenol! Yet, the situation is little better today. Except for drugs, modern "migraineurs" find little hope in the orthodox medical profession for relief or cure. As such, various alternative treatments are often pursued. These include acupuncture, chiropractic, nutrition, homeopathy, osteopathy, biofeedback, physical therapy, massage and even faith healing. For one thing is universal; continue on they must with the hope of finding a cure, as their pain is often so agonizing that they wish to die.

Headache victims cannot be blamed for feeling this way. Why should they lose hope for a cure? Why must they continue having severe migraine attacks for untold numbers of years? There is no reason for continued suffering, because there are answers. Many of these answers are likely right under the person's nose in the form of the food they eat and the beverages they drink.

In respect to chronic illnesses, modern medicine offers few, if any, cures. In regard to migraines, physicians rely primarily upon drugs which are impotent in achieving long-term cures. Medications may be used to abort certain types of headaches and are often useful for relieving the pain. Even so, there are instances where the most potent medications fail to curb headache pain. Plus, there is always the risk of side effects.

Today, migraine has become its own unique disease. Up to 20% of the population is affected. Thus, there are literally millions of sufferers. What's more, each person has developed his/her own unique migraine pattern. Some have migraines on a monthly basis, others by the week, and some unfortunate souls have them every day. Since there are many kinds of headaches, the question might arise: Exactly what constitutes a migraine? This subject will be addressed in the forthcoming chapters.

In the United States headaches cause more pain for more people than any other single condition. Every day approximately 12.5 million Americans suffer from headaches, and a large percentage of these are migraines. Most of these sufferers have the impression that their headaches are largely incurable and that the standard measures of medicine and bed rest are about all that can be done to help cope.

On the contrary there are many answers far superior in curative potential than medication and bed rest. Are these answers biofeedback, stress reduction and psychoanalysis? Not in the least. To cure migraines is to understand them and to uncover the underlying cause. None of the "mental" or anti-stress therapies even begin to approach the cause, at least in the majority of instances.

If stress and emotional problems are not the primary cause, what is the missing factor? Many people overlook the fact that the vast majority of migraine headaches result from physical problems, physical derangements and physical diseases, not mental or psychological ones.

This book makes one simple claim. It is that migraine headaches can be cured *if* the cause is discovered and *if* appropriate treatment is prescribed. In the majority of instances, that cause is food allergies. Undoubtedly, these are strong words. Yet, these statements are based upon years of clinical experience and a great deal of scientific data. Plus, this makes a lot of sense, and common sense is important in the author's view and in the view of many patients as well.

Let it be reiterated that migraine headaches are, for the most part, a curable condition. The sufferer need not live with the pain. Why the repetition? Because most people feel that there are few options to pursue and that they have no choice but to endure the pain. Many have been told by medical professionals that the most which can be done is to treat the symptoms in order to ease the pain. Nearly everyone knows that the primary treatment for migraines is over-the-counter medicine such as aspirin and Tylenol, and millions of dollars of these are sold each month. In severe cases, special drugs like Cafergot, Inderal, Midrin and Valium are prescribed. Some pain-ridden individuals are given injections of potent narcotics like Demerol to gain relief. This is a common prescription in emergency rooms.

In regard to the diagnosis and treatment of migraines, it is important to keep an open mind. The current medical model for treatment is inadequate. The exceptions are those migraines which are due to serious, underlying disease.

There is little scientific proof that medicines aid in the elimination of headaches. Rather, they serve only to treat the symptoms. Aspirin is a good example. Americans consume over 70 billion tablets of aspirin every year, which amounts to a staggering 20 million pills per day. Headache is the number one illness for which aspirin is used. Arthritis is next, with back pain and fever also resulting in significant consumption. Through all this aspirin usage, is the incidence of migraine or arthritis decreasing? No—both diseases are on the rise.

Others use aspirin even though they have no aches or pains. Every day they take it on the supposition that an aspirin a day will keep the doctor away, that is, the cardiovascular surgeon or cardiologist. This is because aspirin thins the blood and may slightly decrease the risk of heart attack and stroke. However, new research indicates that risks for digestive disorders, internal bleeding—including life-threatening intracranial bleeding—and cancer are increased as a result of this daily aspirin intake. This is not surprising, since cardiovascular disease is certainly not caused by an aspirin deficiency. To those who claim vitamins to be a fad is raised the question, "What about aspirin faddism?" The 1990's should truly be given a place in history as the time of the "aspirin epidemic."

Aspirin is not candy. Unfortunately, some children think so. Far from being innocuous, it accounts for more cases of childhood illness and death than any other pill or poison. Plus, it is responsible for the fatal childhood disease known as *Reye's Syndrome*. Why play with fire?

Each year, dozens become ill and many die from aspirin toxicity. The author has personally known of patients who consumed 10 to 20 or more aspirin per day often for several continuous days in order to relieve headache pain. Many who consumed such massive doses suffer physiological damage to this day. In high doses, aspirin damages tissues throughout the body, including the lining of the stomach and intestines, the liver, arteries, veins, brain and kidneys. The immune system is negatively affected and, as is the case with Reye's Syndrome, sometimes irreversibly. Certain adult aspirin users can develop a Reye's-like syndrome involving chronic viral infections—not enough to kill, but enough to debilitate. Such individuals are highly vulnerable to recurrent viral infections as well as to infections by yeasts and parasites.

It becomes clear that aspirin can have a negative effect on virtually any body system. It impairs immunity, damages the intestines, irritates the liver and inflames the kidneys. By all this aspirin-induced trauma, the susceptibility to migraines actually increases.

It is understandable that drugs may be taken to ease the pain. However, this is a temporary measure. It is of more importance to work towards eradicating the problem altogether. Nothing can be more important than that. The migraine sufferer will surely agree. The primary goal of any reasonable treatment plan would be to eliminate the headaches once and for all. At a minimum, the headaches should be reduced in frequency and severity. What could be more important than to be freed, finally, of all the pain, agony, irritability, frustration and all the rest of the sickening feelings? Whatever the symptoms might be, if the cause is treated, they can all disappear.

What choice does the sufferer have, anyway? He/she must pursue any angle possible and cannot afford to be closed-minded. Such an individual has already tried the orthodox medical approach. Often, hopes for a cure have been dashed early in the game, being obliterated by comments such as, "There is no cure for migraine. You'll have to learn to live with it." The desperate patient presses the doctor to check more thoroughly, to try again to find a cause. The doctor will, albeit often reluctantly, run a battery of tests. The patient may be hospitalized to perform the tests which often include sophisticated procedures such as CAT scans, MRI's, brain scans, angiographs and other x-rays. Blood and urine tests are also performed. The hopeful patient awaits the verdict, but invariably the response is, "We checked everything, but all the tests are negative." Oh what despair the patient must feel at that trying moment—the futility of it all: all that time, hope and money in search for a cure, down the drain. Yet, frequently, all the patient was hoping for was an answer, any answer. These patients are willing to accept virtually any verdict—even that of a brain tumor—just to find out once and for all *why all the pain*. Ultimately, the migraine sufferer loses hope and slumps into the continuation of a seemingly endless nightmare—living with excruciating, mind-boggling and sometimes mind-damaging pain.

Can migraines be serious? Can they kill? There is no question that some headaches are caused by life-threatening diseases such as brain tumors, meningitis, blood clots and aneurysms. However, in terms of chronic migraine headaches, these illnesses account for a very small minority. Fortunately, most people reading this book have had the serious causes of headaches ruled out long ago. All that remains is a world of pain without any answers. For that majority this book provides information that, if applied, will change lives forever. It can give the reader a chance to be free of headache pain—once and for all.

CHAPTER 1
What Started All This Pain?

Are you reading this book because you have migraines? If so, was a diagnosis made somewhere along the line? Or, do you just know from the symptoms you experience? In most instances, those who know they have migraines have had the diagnosis confirmed by a physician. Usually, the patterns exhibited by the headache—the distribution of the pain, one side or both, the *prodroma*, a fancy word for the symptoms occurring just prior to the headache's onset, and concurrent symptoms such as nausea, vomiting, visual disturbances, etc., all were considered before the final diagnosis was made.

Even so, many important questions remain. Just what causes the headaches? Or, are there several causes to consider? When did they first begin? For how many years have they existed? How often do they occur? What precipitates them? How long do they last? What makes them worse? What gives them relief? Is there a history of a serious fall or accident? What is the dental history? Is there a family history of migraine and/or food allergy? All these questions must be answered before an accurate assessment can be made and an appropriate treatment prescribed.

Additional questions which are important to discern in the initial history include:

1. Is there a history of a whiplash or other car accident injury occurring prior to the onset of the migraines?

2. Is there a long-term history of lower back trouble?

1

3. Is there a habit of sleeping on the stomach?

4. Does the patient often awaken with a headache?

5. Prior to a headache, does noticeable weight gain or swelling in the extremities occur?

6. If female, is there a history of premenstrual syndrome (PMS)?

7. Are depression, hair loss and/or cold extremities coinciding symptoms?

8. Is there a history of symptoms associated with blood sugar disturbances including irritability, fatigue, mood swings, falling asleep after meals, hyperactivity, mental confusion, depression, anxiety, agitation and digestive disturbances?

9. Is there a history of chronic constipation?

10. Is the patient currently taking blood thinners, blood pressure medicines and/or medications for heart disease?

11. Is there a history of high blood pressure?

12. Is there a history of severe, debilitating viral infections, particularly viral infections of the brain (encephalitis)?

13. Is there a history of lumbar puncture (spinal tap) for surgery or childbirth?

There appears to be some confusion concerning how to classify the severity of migraines. Part of this is due to the bizarre frequency patterns which many headache sufferers experience. There are those whose headaches occur every day. Others experience weekly headaches. Some individuals have headaches that occur every weekend as regularly as clockwork. Still others have monthly or bi-monthly headaches. Then again, the severity of these headaches differs with each case. For these reasons, a unique evaluation method called the Migraine Intensity Exam has been devised. Take this test to see how severely you score.

Migraine Intensity Exam

Which of the following do you experience in regard to migraines either prior to or during the headache?

Points

1. The frequency is best described as:
   a) daily   30
   b) every other day   20

c) twice per week	15
d) once per week	10
e) once per month	5

2. Pain resistant to medication 10

3. Swelling of the extremities, bloating and/or weight gain 10

4. Bloodshot eyes 5

5. Nausea 5

6. Vomiting 10

7. Other digestive disturbances (diarrhea, constipation, stomach pain, etc.) 5

8. Sensitivity to light or sound 5

9. Blurred or impaired vision and/or other visual disturbances 5

10. Numbness of the arm, hand or shoulder preceding the headaches 5

11. Headaches which last over two days 5

Your Score: _____

Scoring

5 to 15 points   *Mild Migraines.* If you scored in this category, you are fortunate. The migraines you experience are mild and infrequent. As such, physical damage is unlikely, and with proper treatment, they should be easily eradicated.

20 to 35 points   *Moderate Migraine Illness.* At this level the migraines are usually severe enough to impair daily activity and to negatively affect lifestyle. One should strive to get rid of them before they worsen or before physical damage occurs.

40 to 55 points   *Severe Migraine Illness.* The consequences of these migraine attacks should be taken seriously. One should do everything possible to find out why they exist, then work towards a plan of reducing their frequency and severity. Usually, the frequency of the headaches can be significantly reduced. In many patients the headaches will be eliminated entirely.

60 and above   *Extremely Severe Migraine Illness.* People in this category have migraines severe enough that tissue damage may result. Most of these patients are taking high doses of medications which further complicate the damage. It is important to immediately determine the cause of the migraines and institute aggressive treatment.

If the reader scores positive for significant migraines, he/she must understand that a "paper diagnosis" is, by itself, insufficient. Laboratory tests must be performed for confirmation.

It is of utmost importance that the patient continues the search for the cause of his/her migraines. This is because the cure can only be achieved once the cause is determined. The practitioner of the healing arts must assist the patient in this effort. There is always a cause. If the physician or practitioner is unable to help, then the responsibility is up to the individual. The remaining chapters will help solve this riddle and put a halt to the endless searching.

CHAPTER 2
Many Kinds, Many Causes

There are many types of headaches. Doctors are taught early in their training to categorize headaches into one of three principal groups: tension headaches, migraine headaches or cluster headaches. Other categories exist, but they are the more rare causes of headaches representing 2% or less of the total headache occurrence. Included are headaches due to blood clots in the brain, traumatic headaches from severe injuries such as concussions, brain infection headaches (meningitis/encephalitis) and the headaches of brain tumor. Headaches related to relatively common medical disorders represent a larger percentage. Diseases and/or illnesses known to produce headaches include high blood pressure, lung disease, hypothyroidism, Cushing's disease, hypoglycemia and infections (fevers). Of note, over one-half of patients with high blood pressure complain of headaches.

In the last 20 years a new category has been added to the list: premenstrual headache. This headache, which is common, occurs either just prior to or during menstruation.

Modern medicine excels in accurate diagnosis of the serious causes of headache. However, it often fails to discern the factors which generate the more common ones. Thus, the cause of tension, migraine, premenstrual and cluster headaches remains elusive and the treatment poor. The majority of headache sufferers are left wandering to and fro between the doctor, hospital, pharmacist, psychiatrist, acupuncturist, chiropractor, physical therapist or masseuse. The approach of modern medicine to chronic headache is probably best exemplified by this quotation from *Harrison's Textbook of Internal Medicine*: "adolescents with daily frontal headaches . . . anxiety or tension is a probable factor. Equally puzzling is the somber, tense adult whose primary complaint is headache, or the migrainous person who in late life or at menopause begins to have daily headaches. *Here it becomes important to assess mental status . . . looking for evidences of anxiety, depression and hypochondriasis.*" In contrast, it can be presumed that anyone with unexplainable chronic headaches or head pain would automatically and understandably become anxious and depressed—or even hypochondriacal—especially if that pain occurred on a daily basis.

Just as there are many kinds of headaches, there are many factors which cause them. As stated previously, there are common and rare causes. All must be considered in the evaluation of headache, although the history should serve as a guide for determining which approach to take. One need not always immediately rush the patient into the x-ray room and impale him/her with cranial x-rays, brain scans and CAT scans at the first sign of a headache. On the other hand, these tools may be invaluable to rule out serious underlying disease. The key is to use good sense, a concept known in medicine as *clinical judgment*. There is another factor. It is peace of mind. It may be necessary to rule out intracranial causes of headaches, including brain tumor, to reassure patients that no such lesion exists, even if the headache fits a "less serious" symptom pattern. Then again, anyone—even the most astute clinician—can be fooled. It is better to be safe than sorry. However, it must be reiterated that the vast majority of headaches are due to causes other than brain tumors. Good judgment is one thing; paranoia is another.

What are these other, less serious causes? There are many, and the most significant ones are listed as follows:

1. allergies to foods and chemicals

2. non-allergic chemical sensitivity

3. structural defects and/or muscle tension

4. hormonal disorders

5. blood sugar disturbances

6. digestive disturbances

7. infections (such as colds and flu)

8. stress

Notice that psychological disorders, such as anxiety and depression, are not listed. This is because mental disorders per se are not a major cause of headaches. Stress does cause headaches. Yet, this occurs by a mechanism which is primarily *physical* in nature, as will be illustrated later in this book.

Look at item Number 1: Allergy. There are literally hundreds of allergic and chemical triggers. As will be discussed in great detail in the next chapter, this appears to be the most common cause. Migraineurs also suffer structural defects, hormonal disturbances and digestive problems. Thus, migraine is more often the result of a combination of several disorders rather than from any single cause. Women with chronic migraines almost always have a combination of allergies plus hormonal problems. As for blood sugar and digestive disturbances, virtually all Americans have them.

Item Number 2, non-allergic chemical sensitivity, represents a significant cause. Categories of chemicals include those which are ingested via food and water, those which are inhaled and those which are contacted and absorbed through the skin.

Fumes are especially likely to trigger headaches, and this occurs for several reasons. Fumes gain direct access to the brain through the nose. At the roof of the nasal cavity is a tiny, thin bony membrane coated with nerves. This region, known as the *cribiform plate*, is the brain's window to the outside world, and it serves the function of being the sensory apparatus for smell. As the brain lies immediately above it, fumes can easily gain direct access through this thin membrane. A "smog headache" can result. There is another mechanism. If the fumes contain carbon monoxide, a highly toxic and potentially lethal gas, the headache can be devastating and prolonged.

Most people are familiar with the cousin of this gas, *carbon dioxide*, which has the chemical formula $CO2$. The chemical formula for carbon monoxide is CO: it is missing an oxygen. This is what makes it so toxic. Upon entering the bloodstream, carbon monoxide seeks oxygen. Where is the most likely place to get it? It is the hemoglobin found in red blood cells, the natural carrier of oxygen. For every molecule of CO inhaled, one molecule of the red blood cell's hemoglobin is neutralized. In essence, carbon monoxide latches onto the hemoglobin molecule and ties up the oxygen so that it cannot be used. This "vice grip" is extremely difficult to break, and the chemical reaction between CO and the red cell is termed in medical textbooks as *irreversible*. This makes it impossible for the red cell to pick up oxygen when it passes by the lungs. One breath of contaminated air leads to the absorption of millions of carbon monoxide molecules. Within minutes most of the body's red cells can be poisoned. The result is oxygen depletion within the tissues to include the number one oxygen consumer, the brain. Fatigue, sleepiness, vague headache and, in the case of prolonged and heavy exposure, death may result.

Here is the point. Headaches may be caused by toxic fumes from a leaky gas stove, a street filled with cars and buses or any other carbon monoxide source which permeates the home or business. Formaldehyde, diesel fumes, car exhaust, sulfur dioxide, chlorine gas and many other gaseous compounds are also known to provoke or aggravate headaches.

While only a comparatively few gases exist, there are hundreds and even thousands of chemicals which can cause headaches. The role played by food additives in migraine causation will be described in detail in the next chapter. It is appropriate to list here the industrial, commercial and agricultural chemicals which can generate a toxic headache:

Industrial/Commercial

Kerosene
Gasoline
Benzene
Dioxin
Carbon Tetrachloride
Fluoride
Industrial cleaners

Bromine (or its gas)
Formaldehyde (or its gas)
Chlorine (or its gas)
Paints and paint fumes
Solvents
PCB's

Agricultural

Nitrates and Nitrites
Pesticides
Herbicides
Fungicides
Fumigants

This list is far from comprehensive. Yet, it does provide a glimpse into how and why headaches are largely a result of our environment. The number of headaches we get may depend to a large degree on how toxic that environment is.

Heavy Metals

Heavy metal toxicity is a common cause of chronic illness in industrialized countries. Since the turn of the century, levels of aluminum, mercury, cadmium, arsenic, lead and nickel have increased in our food and water by several hundred percent. One of the most frequent symptoms of heavy metal toxicity is headache. This is especially true of lead, copper and mercury poisoning.

Heavy metal poisoning should always be ruled out as a potential cause of chronic headaches. Research indicates that copper can provoke a certain type of migraine by interfering with the transmission of nerve impulses in the brain. However, the same is true of mercury and lead, since both have a high affinity for nerve tissues and are, therefore, likely to disrupt the function of the brain and spinal nerves. Thus, the chronic headaches of heavy metal poisoning are actually due to heavy metal overload of the brain. An excellent screen for heavy metal exposure is hair analysis (see Chapter Three).

Drugs and Other Chemicals

It is true that many synthetic chemicals can provoke headaches, but so can certain natural chemicals. Cigarette smoke, ergotamine, aflatoxin, biological amines (found in wines and cheeses), alkaloids (found in herbs and spices) and nitrates are examples of naturally occurring toxins capable of initiating headaches.

Certain drugs cause headaches. Most notable are birth control pills (BCP's) which are commonly used. The pill is not only a potent cause of headaches, but it also aggravates existing migraine conditions. Other drugs known to cause headaches include cortisone, Indocin, aspirin, Cardiazem, Tylenol, Coumadin and Hydralazine. In addition, megadoses of vitamin A over a prolonged period can cause headaches. Note that two of the most common agents used to treat migraine, aspirin and Tylenol, can actually cause it. This response can be due to an allergy to the drug. Thus, if a person is sensitive to aspirin or Tylenol, taking it during a migraine will act to prolong the attack and may even make the pain worse.

Many drugs which lower blood pressure also cause headaches. This is due to a reduction in blood flow to the brain. Diuretics operate via this mechanism, although they also cause deficiencies of anti-headache minerals such as potassium, calcium and magnesium.

Cigarette smoke is a common cause of headaches both in smokers and in passive inhalers. One study performed in Britain showed that over 50% of smokers became headache free just by quitting. No doubt this indicates that smokers are allergic to the tobacco leaf and also to the smoke that is generated from it. For BCP users, similar results are seen with over 30% becoming headache free after discontinuing the pill.

The Role of Stress

Many people assume that headaches are a result of stress. Others know of no obvious stressor that provokes them, rather, believing that the stress they experience is due to headaches. In reality, both of these beliefs hold some truth. There is no question that stress can and does bring on headaches.

One important question is, what are the mechanisms by which stress can induce headaches? Mental stress initiates a wide array of physical responses. Both physical and mental stress weaken a person's defenses. Whenever an individual is stressed, strain is placed upon internal organs such as the immune system, digestive tract, liver, thyroid and adrenals. This strain is mediated via the central nervous system (CNS), the region first affected by stress. The CNS sends nerve impulses in response to our thoughts to the various organs and glands. Positive thoughts result in the delivery of useful impulses, and negative thoughts deliver harmful ones.

The ill effects of stress differ from person to person. Everyone is subjected to it every day. Our thoughts can either neutralize or aggravate these unavoidable stresses. It is important to minimize the ill effects of stress as much as possible. In order to do so, it is helpful to study some of the natural anti-stress mechanisms.

When the mind entertains a stressful thought, numerous physiological reactions begin to occur. Impulses arising in the brain are delivered directly to the internal organs through the spinal cord and peripheral nerves. The stomach responds with the secretion of hydrochloric acid. The liver responds by synthesizing sugar, or, as is the case in chronic stress, by increasing the synthesis of cholesterol. The adrenal glands react by increasing the production of adrenalin and other adrenal hormones. The pancreas pumps out more insulin, and the thyroid increases metabolism through the synthesis of additional thyroid hormone. The thymus, that all-important immune gland located behind the sternum, shrinks in response to stress.

Stress, Blood Sugar and Migraine

What does all this mean in terms of migraines? One effect is predictable: a drop in blood sugar levels. The brain is highly sensitive to its energy needs and is dependent upon glucose, the primary sugar in the blood, for that energy. A sudden drop in blood sugar levels, a common end result of stress, negatively affects the brain. Often, the result is a variety of symptoms which may include severe pain and migraine. It is important to note that the adrenal glands are damaged by stress. This is significant, since they are involved in blood sugar control. Whether the adrenal abuse is due to physical or mental stress, the end result is the same: an increase in the secretion of adrenal hormones resulting in either a sudden drop in blood sugar levels or the inability to maintain adequate levels. Eventually, as a consequence of over-production, the adrenal glands are no longer able to produce adequate amounts of hormones. This subject will be discussed in greater detail in Chapter Five.

Both the pancreas and the liver help manage blood sugar levels. The pancreas is especially important, since it produces insulin. This is the primary hormone for regulating blood sugar levels. Stress often leads to the production of excess amounts of insulin. The combination of the stress-induced secretion of adrenal hormones and insulin into the bloodstream can be a double whammy to the brain. This is because too much of a good thing—an excess of these hormones—causes blood sugar levels to drop suddenly. When the brain is deprived of glucose, which is its primary fuel, a headache often results.

Stress also leads to muscular tension. Put simply, stress tightens and places torque upon the joints and muscles. Muscle spasm often results, and this spasm leads to pressure upon the nerves themselves. The pressure causes pain, and the result is headache. This is descriptively known as *tension headache*. Often, many migraines are a combination of true migraine plus tension headache.

What is most interesting about stress-induced headaches is that, often, if the underlying problems are corrected, the headaches go away *even if the stress remains the same.* Even so, it is advised that stressed individuals learn new ways to better cope with their problems. There is nothing good about stress. All it does is damage. Sometimes it even kills.

Intestinal Reflexes

Could an irritant in the stomach or intestines cause a headache? Experience and research prove that it can. There is a special relationship between the head and gut, a relationship maintained by the vagus nerve.

The vagus is classified as a cranial nerve. This means that it arises within the brain and exits directly from the skull without going into the spinal cord. It is the main nerve supply to the stomach, intestines, liver, pancreas and colon. Along the way the vagus divides into several branches, including some in the neck.

The vagus is a powerful nerve. When it becomes irritated, it can produce a variety of symptoms. One of them is head pain. How does this occur? The vagus is not a pain nerve per se. What does result is a form of referred pain known medically as *vagal cephalalgia*. This term defines scalp pain and/or headaches of vagal origin. It only stands to reason that if the cause of the vagus nerve irritation is shut off, the pain will recede. For instance, if the stomach is inflamed, nerve fibers arising from it may refer pain to the scalp, particularly the scalp on top of the head. If the inflammation is treated with agents specific for stomach disorders such as ginger or licorice root, the head pain often disappears.

A more dramatic example occurs within the colon. It too contains vagal nerve fibers which, when irritated, produce referred pain. In this case pain may be on the top of the head and also quite often in the rear or occipital region.

The most common cause of *colonic cephalalgia* is constipation. A plugged up bowel can cause headaches simply by increasing mechanical pressure on colonic nerves. When the pressure is released, as occurs with a healthy bowel movement, the headache or head pain dramatically goes away. Some believe that constipation causes headaches primarily by intoxication, that is, the pollution of the blood by one's own waste. While this can occur, constipation headaches are more commonly due to mechanical factors. This was proven by Dr. Alvarez of the Mayo Clinic. He reproduced headaches in susceptible patients by stuffing cotton in their rectums.

A great deal can be done to prevent constipation headaches. Here are some useful measures:

1. Answer the call of nature whenever it occurs. Avoid "holding it." Go when you need to go. This is a most critical factor.

2. Go for a walk every day. The best anti-constipation exercise is a brisk walk in the morning before or after breakfast. The walk should be a minimum of 1/2 mile, although 1 to 2 miles is preferable.

3. Drink 6 large glasses of water daily (non-chlorinated) and eat water-retaining foods. Such foods retain moisture in the colon, and this creates stools which are bulky and soft. A partial list of these foods includes:

watermelon	carrots
cantaloupe	lettuce
honeydew melon	celery
citrus fruits	parsley
kiwi	pea pods
grapes	water chestnuts
apples	turnips
pears	watercress
tomatoes	onions
cucumbers	spinach
eggplant	squash
cabbage	radishes
endive	

4. Take supplemental fiber sources. The extra fiber should be consumed daily. Good sources of fiber include:

   - bran, especially oat, corn, wheat, barley and rice*
   - psyllium husk and seed
   - alfalfa
   - fruit pectin
   - vegetable fibers

5. Take an acidophilus supplement. This will add to the bulk of the stool and assist in easing elimination.

To become educated about all the various types of headaches is important. However, it is difficult for the headache patient to pin down precisely what might be causing his/her headaches without medical help. This issue will be addressed in the next chapter.

* Many people are allergic to grains and, in these cases, other less allergenic sources of fiber must be used.

CHAPTER 3
Making the Diagnosis

Headache sufferers face a major dilemma. Their pain is real—this they know. To be rid of the pain is their goal, one which they pursue with great deliberation. Usually, they have no clue as to what brings on the headaches. To complicate matters, the medical profession has difficulty finding any answers, unless a diagnosis of organic disease can be made. For the most part, medical doctors or, for that matter, other health professionals such as chiropractors, osteopathic physicians, acupuncturists and dentists, really have no idea what to do. They may wish to help the patient but often find that they have few directions in which to turn. This chapter has been designed for these doctors and for concerned patients. Common sense dictates that migraines have a biological cause. It is likely that many health practitioners will agree with this and wish to learn all they can about innovative methods for treating this pervasive illness.

An engineer must first determine the source of a bridge weakness before he can rebuild it. A TV repairman must find out why a unit is on the blink before it can be fixed. An auto mechanic must make a diagnosis concerning a defective engine before he can begin repairs. The same should hold true in the medical field. Such was the philosophy of Andrew Taylor Still, M.D., the founder of Osteopathic Medicine who said in relation to human illness, "Find it, fix it and leave it alone."

Modern or Western medicine is one of the few medical systems which treats symptoms instead of causes. Both East Indian and Chinese medicine attempt to search for the cause. The ancient Greeks made a partial attempt to get to the bottom of things, though their system was greatly

13

improved during the Middle Ages by Arab/Persian doctors who were thorough cause-seekers. American Indian medicine was cause-oriented as were some of the medicinal approaches of South American societies such as the Incas.

The American Indians, the original inhabitants of North and South America, were a people in tune with nature. In the realm of the healing arts, they utilized naturally occurring substances—foods, food extracts and herbs. Often, they administered highly specific therapies in their attempts to cure illness. Many of these remedies are only now being recognized for their curative potential.

If this has been man's historical tendency, why is there such a deficiency of this philosophy in the current forms of medicine? If anything, we should be further advanced in using the scientific method to determine cause and effect. Considering the advancements of modern science, the determination of what is causing a given person's headaches, and, the accomplishment of its final cure should be a rapid, efficient and effective process. This should be the status quo.

Instead, the patient with migraine is often confronted with a barrage of futile questions and/or undergoes a battery of inconclusive tests. All too often the medical effort amounts to little more than a random attempt to reassure the concerned patient that, "Nothing serious is wrong." Once all the obvious medical causes are ruled out, the frustrated physician may proclaim, "It's all in your head" or "You're under too much stress." As a result, the unfortunate soul is often referred to a psychiatrist. Some people are even blamed for their headaches—as if they created them on purpose! The scenario is something like this, "You are holding onto your pain for some emotional reason." This is just so much nonsense. It is important to avoid taking these comments personally, as the doctor is probably so frustrated that he/she just doesn't know what else to do. The tipoff to this medical frustration is the question, "Are you having personal problems?" You can imagine what the next suggestion will be.

Stalling and making excuses is nothing new in the professions. Doctors and lawyers do it. Accountants are known to stall. Husbands do it to wives, and visa versa. Even kids know the art of stalling. In fact, they are probably better at it than anyone else. Why is this important? Because it is crucial for the migraine sufferer to make a distinction and to know the difference between someone who can help them and someone who is only biding time.

The physician must be aggressive at determining the underlying cause of migraine. He/she should perform a thorough history and physical examination and run the appropriate tests if any are indicated. Usually, doctors lean towards the philosophy that the history is the most important part of any evaluation. While this is true of many diseases, there is a special variation that applies to patients with chronic migraines. As a rule, the most important step in diagnosing and curing migraines is laboratory testing. This means that tests are more revealing in achieving a migraine cure than are the history and physical.

However, it must be noted that a thorough history and complete physical exam are mandatory in any migraine evaluation. Great care must be taken to insure that the headaches are not due to serious or life-threatening disease, and a thorough history and physical are the best ways to do this.

Through these three methods—the history, the physical and the tests—the sufferer can usually find out whether his/her worst fears are true. Is there any hope? Are the headaches simply a result of stress, or is there an underlying cause? Are the migraines a consequence of serious and life-threatening disease, or is the problem a simple and curable one? Are the headaches a result of psychological disturbances, or are they simply the manifestation of a malingering hypochondriac? Many migraine patients have been so labeled.

How to Make a Diagnosis

Headaches can be a symptom of serious, underlying disease. Most people are aware of the life-threatening causes of headaches such as brain tumors, cancer, stroke, aneurysms, cerebral hemorrhage and meningitis. Many of these conditions are associated with a sudden onset of symptoms, although a few, such as certain brain tumors, can exhibit symptoms over a prolonged period. These symptoms might include severe pain, headache, nausea, vomiting, dizziness, loss of consciousness, extremely stiff neck and visual loss. Such symptoms, especially if acute or following injury, require medical diagnosis and treatment. It is possible that certain people will become overly concerned by this statement, since some of the mentioned symptoms occur in migraines of less serious origin. Fortunately, most migraine sufferers have long since had these serious conditions ruled out. For that majority, other less ominous disorders must be held responsible.

Types of Tests

There are six major categories of tests useful for evaluating migraines. They are as follows:

1. *Tests to rule out serious causes.* These include CAT scans, MRI's, brain scans, x-rays, EEG's, angiographs and certain blood tests.

2. *Food allergy testing.* The recommended test involves highly sophisticated, specialized blood testing for immune-allergy reactions to numerous foods.

3. *Vitamin/mineral assessment.* This is done primarily through blood, hair and urine analysis.

4. *Digestive analysis.* This is done via blood, urine and stool assays.

5. *Hormonal gland function.* This is accomplished through high-tech blood and urine analysis.

6. *Toxic Metal Analysis.* This is done primarily through analyzing hair or tissue samples, although blood and urine samples are occasionally used.

These tests can be utilized to diagnose most migraines. For the majority of patients, tests in the first category will be negative. Nearly all will have significant allergies, and many will test positive for nutritional deficiencies, digestive disturbances and hormonal dysfunction.

One of the last stages in establishing the diagnosis is selecting the medical terminology. Everyone is interested in knowing his/her diagnosis. According to the system promulgated in this book, the chronic migraine sufferer will rarely qualify for only one diagnosis. The typical case is something like this: MIGRAINE HEADACHE, HYPOTHYROIDISM, FOOD ALLERGIES and INTESTINAL MALABSORPTION. Other diagnoses commonly determined in migraine patients include adrenal cortical insufficiency, intestinal parasites, anemia, thyroiditis, hypotension, carbohydrate intolerance and hypertension.

Finally, it is necessary for both the chronically ill and the health practitioner to have goals. The prime objective should be to eliminate the headaches. This is possible in the majority of cases. In a few instances, the best that can be accomplished is to reduce the severity and frequency of the migraines so that life can become more normal. As with anything in life, persistence pays off.

There are millions of people whose lives are strapped by migraine and migraine pain. Headaches draw the fun out of life. They drain vitality and impair productivity. Just as the blood flow stagnates in the victims' brains, so do their lives. Every day with its pains and frustrations is a potentially useful day lost. The headache sufferer knows this all too well.

Making a diagnosis is not difficult. All the tools are available. Any physician can do it. Unfortunately, patients are at the mercy of a medical profession inadequately informed about the causation of disease. Finding a physician who is willing to pursue these angles or who has the expertise to do so is often a difficult task. A small list of physicians, medical institutions and chiropractors capable of assisting the migraineur is provided in Appendix D. Chiropractors, while unable to perform many of the more sophisticated medical tests, are allowed to draw blood in certain states and are skilled in some of the structural therapies described in this book. The ideal, of course, would be to find a D.O. or an M.D. skilled in these techniques.

Migraine sufferers are in pain, and they desire relief. Making the diagnosis helps stop this on-going crisis by:

1. Giving the patient some hard answers, including medical diagnoses illustrating the cause.

2. Providing patients with hope for a cure.

3. Helping migraineurs to be more accurate observers. The more knowledge they have about what triggers their headaches, the easier it is to avoid them.

4. Giving both the physician and patient direction so that a cure can be efficiently accomplished.

Hope is in and despair is out. Bernie Siegel recommends it. Norman Cousins espoused it. Wayne Dyer demands it. These are learned men. Listening to the hopeless is picking the wrong company, especially when it comes to migraine headaches. If a diagnosis can be determined, there is hope. Odds are, there is also a cure.

CHAPTER 4
Allergies: The Number One Cause

Allergies are the missing link in the mystery of migraine causation. What is most intriguing is that more migraines are caused by allergies to naturally occurring substances than by all those caused by synthetics, chemicals, drugs and fumes combined. It is actually food allergies that are the main culprit. This includes allergies to natural beverages such as coffee or tea. This may be difficult for many people to believe, but it is true. Very few people—whether lay person or professional—are aware of this food allergy-migraine connection. How could food, the nourishment for our survival, cause headaches? How can something natural and wholesome cause misery and pain? The mechanisms for how this occurs are now well understood. Modern researchers have found that foods are made up of a complexity of compounds, many of which can cause the reactions leading to headaches.

The concept that food allergy is the major force in causing migraines is far from a new medical discovery. Rather, it was known as early as 1907 that food allergies cause migraines. In 1936, Goltman wrote a monumental research paper entitled, "Mechanism of Migraine." In this article, he reported a case of a patient who was mistakenly subjected to brain surgery during a migraine crisis. The operation was performed during the migraine attack, and the surgeons were able to directly view what occurred. It was observed that the patient's brain and brain membranes were markedly swollen and inflamed, but no serious abnormality or disease was found.

Several days later, it was determined that the patient was allergic to wheat. Amazingly, when the patient was challenged with wheat, similar swelling was palpable. This was easy to determine, since the surgery left a temporary opening in the skull.

The link between migraines and food allergies was largely neglected until the 1950's when Doctors Leon Unger and Joel Cristol, both M.D.'s, wrote their landmark article entitled "Allergic Migraine." This article appeared in the prominent medical journal for allergists, *Annals of Allergy.* The gist of the article is best described by these authors' own words: "Migraine is an allergic disease due to one or more foods." This is a profound statement. The medical profession is either unaware of this finding or chooses to remain ignorant of it. In case it has been a matter of oversight, there is no reason for medical professionals to remain oblivious of this data as well as the plethora of the more modern data offering the same conclusions. Migraine patients have suffered too much and too long for no good reason. The irony is the answers have been there all along. For instance, in an article published in 1921 in the *Journal of the American Medical Association*, Dr. Brown claimed that diet played a role in migraines. In 1930, Dr. LaRoche and colleagues noted that foods cause migraine. Dr. Theron Randolph, a medical doctor and allergist of the modern era, has been espousing this for years and has written several books and research articles on the subject.

Numerous articles have recently been published in major medical journals denoting the current views on migraine and food allergy. Many of these articles are listed in the bibliography of this book. The conclusion is the same: *Migraine is caused by food allergy, food allergy and food allergy until proven otherwise.*

For those who would like to argue the point, consider this; What harm would come to the patient if it is presumed that he/she experiences migraines due to food allergy? Wouldn't it be worth a try to treat migraines with this in mind and see what happens? Even if no improvement is registered, at least no harm will be done. This is the minimum amount of care that should be attempted. Instead, the migraine patient is often bluntly told, "Diet and allergies have nothing to do with headaches."

The Migraine Personality: Does it Really Exist?

Most psychologists and psychiatrists, as well as many physicians, believe in what is called the *migraine personality.* This stereotype is thought to occur commonly in women, especially menstruating women, but it also may be ascribed to men. The women are supposedly perfectionists who are obsessed with keeping everything in order to the tiniest detail at work or home. As this theory goes, the perfectionism causes emotional stress which provokes migraines. Another female stereotype is the *hypochondriac.* A hypochondriac is defined as a person who complains of an illness which does not exist. According to this theory, migraineurs use their illness to accomplish everything from seeking attention to expressing anger over a forlorn relationship. In my experience, nothing could be further from the truth. In fact, I have yet to see a single case of the migraine personality. This experience is not isolated. In the words of Dr. Unger, whose outstanding research is regarded as a landmark in migraine causation, "Although emotions can precipitate attacks, *it is only in those who are allergic to one or more foods*" [italics mine]. It was reasonable for Dr. Unger to feel this way, since over 90% of his migraine patients showed either significant improvement or complete eradication of their headaches once the allergic foods were omitted from their diets. Some of the most solid research on the food allergy-migraine connection was done by Dr. Unger in 1952 at which time he found that there are three types of migraines: 1) Those caused exclusively by foods. 2) Those in which foods appear to play a minor role. 3) Those caused by foods under certain conditions, including stress or exhaustion. Dr. Unger also discovered that certain chemicals, including food additives, cause migraines. Some of the more common chemical agents that he determined to be migraine provokers are as follows:

- alcohol
- nitrates (and nitrites)
- caffeine
- phenylethylamine
- tyramine

- monosodium glutamate (MSG)
- theobromine
- benzoic acid
- food dyes
- salicylates

The Allergy-Migraine Connection: A Review of Scientific Literature

Since the early 1950's, numerous articles have been written concerning the food allergy, food additive and chemical connection with migraines. Here are some of the key findings discussed in these articles:

1. Mansfield and associates, in a study involving 43 adult migraine sufferers, reduced headache frequency by two thirds by removing suspected allergic foods from the diet.

2. Dr. Vaughan found that nearly one half of patients with chronic migraine were aided, in terms of a reduction in the frequency and severity of their headaches, when foods such as eggs, milk, corn and wheat were eliminated from the diet.

3. As early as 1921, researchers found chemicals in the blood of migraine patients which constricted arteries within the brain, leading to pain. Later it was found that these substances, serotonin and histamine, are the very chemicals which are liberated during allergic reactions.

4. Recently, it was discovered that migraine sufferers' platelets are more

sticky than normal. These platelets clog circulation and may also release serotonin and other chemicals which are associated with the genesis of headache pain. It has long been known that allergic reactions cause platelets to become activated and "clump" together.

5. Dr. Mansfield found that certain foods commonly cause migraines. These foods include milk, wheat, corn, egg, soybean, peanut, chocolate and alcoholic beverages. He determined that eliminating these foods led to an improvement in the majority of cases.

6. In 1989, researchers at the Montefiore Medical Headache Unit in New York found that out of a total of 171 patients, approximately 50% reported alcohol as a precipitating factor for migraines. Nearly 10% associated Nutra Sweet as a trigger.

7. Dr. Ellen Grant of the Department of Neurology, Charing Cross Hospital, London, England, achieved a significant reduction in migraines via allergy removal. Of the 60 patients tested, 50 became headache free, an 85% improvement. What's more, an unexpected benefit was seen. Of the 15 patients who had high blood pressure, all had normal blood pressure by the end of the study.

8. Concerning a concept first described by Rowe in 1931, it has been found that many people have allergies without realizing it and without obvious symptoms. The only way that an individual can experience a reaction to a hidden allergy is to eliminate the food from the diet for several weeks and then reintroduce it. Only then can obvious symptoms due to the food be produced. Chronic illnesses, including migraines, were found to be caused by these hidden food allergies.

9. Dr. Monro and her colleagues found that two-thirds of severe migraine sufferers had food allergies and that these allergies were the primary cause of their headaches. This allergy-migraine connection was determined by a combination of allergy testing and food avoidance. The results of this study were reported in 1980 in the prominent British medical journal, *The Lancet*.

10. For years, researchers have known that the risks of internal bleeding within the brain are greatly increased in users of birth control pills. Women who use the pill are 6 times more likely to develop cerebral bleeding and, if they also smoke, they are 22 times more likely. Based upon the pill's adverse effects upon cerebral circulation, Dr. Ellen Grant felt an investigation of its effects upon migraine was warranted. The results were as would be expected. Women on the pill had 3 times as many migraines as non-users, and it was determined that these pill-induced migraines can be both severe and damaging. Dr. Grant recorded the existence of actual tissue damage to arteries and veins within the brain. She also found that small arteries, known as

arterioles, found within the pain-sensitive uterus were thicker in BCP users than non-users. Another abnormality was that the uterine veins were swollen and congested.

It would appear that evidence is accumulating that birth control pills are more toxic than the public has been led to believe. Dr. Grant feels that this toxicity is largely due to a bizarre alteration in liver function.

11. In 1983, Dr. J. Egger and fellow researchers presented findings on the cause of childhood migraine which were published in a prominent British medical journal. This research was performed at the Hospital for Sick Children and Institute of Child Health in London, England. Their findings are summarized as follows: 93% of children with severe migraines recovered completely with no further headaches when allergic foods were identified and removed. What's more, other complaints and illnesses including asthma, behavioral disorders, stomach pain and eczema were also improved or were eliminated.

By summarizing these findings, a point has been made. These are legitimate, scientific studies performed by experienced researchers. In addition, all of these studies were published in prominent medical journals. The evidence is clear: migraine headaches and food allergy are inseparable.

I have successfully treated over 50 cases of chronic migraine which only further solidifies the truth of what these researchers have determined. Many of these patients have searched far and wide for a cure. Nearly half experienced migraines for greater than 15 years. Yet, all are either cured or considerably improved. The researchers quoted previously had similar dramatic results. Physicians who read this book should take note of one fact: patients who have migraines want to be rid of their problem. If the physician wishes to serve a useful function in regard to the migraine patient, he/she must become familiarized with the role food allergies play in causing migraines.

One physician cannot possibly see all the migraine patients who exist. Therefore, it is the aim of this book to provide both the lay person and the professional with convincing data that alternative therapies for migraines exist and that they are highly effective. The public desperately needs more open-minded, nutritionally oriented practitioners. It is difficult to find such physicians in a major metropolitan area, let alone more rural regions or medium-sized cities. However, the awareness of the value of preventive and nutritional medicine is increasing. Physicians who specialize in the diagnosis of food allergy through the method described in this book are listed in Appendix D. Unfortunately, the doctors listed are found only in a few states, notably the Midwest. Hopefully, by the time of the next printing, other listings will be included.

Almost any food or beverage can cause migraines. Does this sound overwhelming? It could be, if you were to attempt to determine the allergies on your own. This is a difficult, time-consuming and inaccurate method for diagnosing food allergies. The easiest way to isolate allergic foods is to utilize diagnostic allergy testing.

It is interesting that many migraineurs who believe they have allergies think they have an awareness of what their allergies are. This is highly unlikely. Why would anyone want to rack his/her brain trying to figure out the allergic foods, especially when the technology exists to find out precisely what these food allergies are? This point is stressed, because many patients resist the idea that they might have hidden food allergies that could cause migraines. When confronted with the prospect that allergies could be involved, they often proclaim, "I already know what my allergies are." Or they state, "Since I don't have any allergy symptoms, I must not have allergies." Both thoughts are erroneous in terms of science and in respect to migraine tendencies. One can be entirely free of common allergy symptoms such as runny nose, hives, itching and rash but still have numerous allergies. I have yet to meet a migraine sufferer who truly knew even a few of his/her allergies, let alone comprehend them all. If such people really knew what their allergies were, they wouldn't have migraines, would they? There are a few exceptionally perceptive individuals who have linked an occasional headache to its cause. Yet, even with these rare people, the origins of the majority of their headaches still elude them.

The Food Intolerance Test—A Simple Method for Determining Migraine-Provoking Foods

Many migraine patients have undergone allergy testing, but they still have migraines. Others have never had an allergy test. In either case, the Food Intolerance Test can prove to be a real boon.

By determining the causative allergies, this test has saved innumerable migraine patients from continual pain and suffering. It is best described as a specialized blood test for diagnosing food, chemical and beverage allergies, and it is perhaps the easiest of all allergy tests to perform. All that is required is the drawing of a single tube of blood done as a fasting sample. What supersedes its simplicity is its accuracy which measures up to 80%. By comparison, scratch testing is 30% to 40% accurate, while RAST testing (for foods) is only about 5% to 15% accurate. The ELISA test, a complex blood test which is relatively new, has been highly touted. However, its accuracy is less than 50%, and only a comparatively few foods are included in the evaluation.

There is yet another allergy testing method. This is fasting followed by a rotation diet. This method has become popular over the last 20 years. It was pioneered by the respected allergist Theron Randolph, M.D. The idea is to go on a complete fast for 3 to 5 days to clear out all reactive compounds from the body. Then, on an empty stomach, suspect foods are introduced one at a time. The patient awaits a measurable reaction such as runny nose, rash, irritability, headache, diarrhea, fatigue, etc. If such symptoms occur, the food is deemed responsible. This is an honorable method. However, it has its limitations. By this method it would take nearly a year to investigate the 200 to 250 foods and food additives commonly found in the diet. The cycle of fasting and adding back of foods would have to be repeated over and over again. In addition, delayed reactions of up to three to four days after food consumption make it difficult to pinpoint the offending food/beverage.

The Food Intolerance Test solves these dilemmas. Overall, its advantages are as follows:

1) It is simple to perform

2) It is accurate.

3) It has a proven track record—hundreds of migraine patients have already benefited

4) It is cost effective

In terms of price, the Food Intolerance Test is truly a value for the money. The cost is approximately $2.00 per food. By comparison, RAST testing costs $8.00 to $12.00 per food, and ELISA runs a minimum of $6.00. Scratch testing may be even more costly.

How the Test is Performed

The test is performed by drawing blood in a special tube which contains a unique preservative. This preservative keeps the human blood cells alive during storage and transport. Once received, the blood is mixed with food extracts. Through a special high-powered microscope, the technician views the interactions and physiological changes that occur within the blood as a result of the food antigen-immune reactions and records them according to severity. Reactions are graded 1, 2 or 3, with 3 being most severe.

A variety of observations are made depending upon the intensity of the immunological reactions. A list of the possibilities include:

1) inflammation

2) clumping of red blood cells

3) clumping of platelets

4) damage to cell membranes

5) reduction in white blood cell mobility

6) destruction of white blood cells

Severe allergic reactions can be associated with inflammation, cell damage and even cell death. It is a sure bet that the same processes occur in the living state as well. Remember, this test is done on *live cells*. It takes little imagination to understand why such allergy reactions produce migraines. Experience with patients proves that mild, moderate and severe reactions all can cause headaches. Sometimes, a person can eat a food to which he/she is mildly allergic without having a headache. However, on other occasions, a migraine is provoked. Perhaps this is an indication of how stressed an individual's system might be on any given day. A person's stress can vary by the hour, by the minute or even by the second.

How Food Allergy Reactions Occur: The Immune Connection

Once it was thought that nearly all allergies were the result of immune reactions against proteins. These proteins are known immunologically as *antigens*. While it is true that protein or antigen-immune reactions account for many allergic responses, it is now known that a variety of allergic reactions can occur as a result of ingesting foods or chemicals devoid of protein. Examples of non-protein substances which can evoke allergy include alcohol, sugar, corn syrup, sulfites, alkaloids, Nutra Sweet and saccharin.

It must be stressed that the protein-antigen reaction mechanism remains a common and extremely important cause of allergic illness. Let's examine how this reaction occurs.

High protein foods are complex compounds made up of untold numbers of protein molecules bound together by molecular bonds. Take a fish fillet, for example. Its useful nutritional components must be liberated by digestive juices in the stomach and intestines. The pancreas secretes potent enzymes which, along with the hydrochloric acid of the stomach, act to break proteins into simpler compounds. Proper function of this digestive process is critical in order to remain healthy.

The tendency to develop allergic reactions to protein is directly related to how thoroughly it is digested. Sluggish or impaired digestion leads to the incomplete breakdown of food.

It was once thought that protein could be absorbed only if it was completely digested into its component parts known as *amino acids*. This theory held that only amino acids could be transported from the intestines into the bloodstream; larger molecules were supposedly prohibited from entry. Now it is known that this theory is wrong. Hundreds of scientific papers have demonstrated that incompletely digested protein molecules, literally undigested food, can be absorbed into the blood and that such proteins greatly increase the vulnerability to food intolerance and immune attack. In migraine this is precisely what occurs; the inappropriately digested protein is regarded as a foreign substance and is attacked by the immune defenses.

White blood cells surround these proteins in order to digest and detoxify them. The immune system also reacts by producing special anti-allergy proteins known as *immunoglobulins*. Several types of immunoglobulins exist. They are known by the abbreviations IgG, IgM, IgD, IgE and IgA. Of these the most important, in terms of allergic defenses, are IgE, IgG and IgA.

In respect to chronic food allergy, IgG and IgA are most important. They are produced by special white blood cells known as *B-lymphocytes*. These lymphocytes are located throughout the body, but heavy concentrations are found within the intestinal walls, in lymph nodes and within the spleen and liver. As such, the B-lymphocytes are strategically located for intercepting bacteria, viruses, yeasts, parasites or allergens—anything which might illicit an immune response. Plus, the B-cells are *immuno-specific*. This means that they will produce a different immunoglobulin for each immune stimulus. Thus, there are anti-bacterial, anti-viral, anti-yeast, anti-parasitic and, yes, anti-food immunoglobulins. In the utterly astounding complexities of human function, there can theoretically be a different immunoglobulin for every food and/or each microbe. In reality, this does not occur. No one is allergic or sensitized to everything. What does occur is that for every food to which an individual is allergic, there is a separate, specific anti-food immunoglobulin being produced.

Just what function do these immunoglobulins perform? They actually attach themselves to—in a sense, surround—the noxious agent which could be protein, food, chemical or microbial. This results in the formation of an *antigen-antibody complex*. These are also known as *immune complexes*. Studies have determined that in migraine sufferers, immune complexes can be found in the arteries of the brain, along the brain membranes, in the arteries of the neck and scalp as well as in seemingly remote organs such as the liver, kidney and uterus. The common medium is the blood which carries these immune complexes and deposits them virtually everywhere. To put it simplistically, the immune system will respond to improperly digested and allergic foods as if they are enemies and will launch a systemic attack. One of the remnants of that attack are the immune complexes.

An important element in preventing allergic reactions is to keep potential allergens from entering the bloodstream. One way to accomplish this is to determine what the allergies are and avoid them. However, what is most interesting is that the human body has developed its own special police force for preventing blood-borne food/chemical reactions. The key player in this force is a special immunoglobulin known as *secretory IgA*. It is so named because it is secreted within the intestinal tract. It is found throughout the entire intestinal canal, including the small intestine, colon, stomach, esophagus and even the mouth. Secretory IgA (S-IgA) is produced in large quantities, some 3,000 to 5,000 milligrams being synthesized per day. Most allergic persons secrete less S-IgA than normal, and some secrete virtually none at all.

Secretory IgA is the First Line of Defense

Secretory IgA is a critical player in the immune defense against allergy. What makes it the front line defender is its strategic position. Normally, this immunoglobulin is formidably poised in high concentrations along the mucous membranes of the intestinal canal. The digestive membranes are the first place where allergic reactions occur, and it is often here that significant chemical and immunological reactions develop. Reactions which occur in the bloodstream are an indication that noxious agents have penetrated the S-IgA front line defense. The critical importance of S-IgA must be stressed, since it blocks the absorption of harmful substances before they gain entry into the blood or lymph. However, if a noxious agent does get by, all is not lost. Internal organs such as the liver, spleen and lymph nodes also contain IgA, as does the blood itself.

Secretory IgA binds to various compounds so these compounds can be neutralized and essentially rendered non-toxic. Also, this binding sends a signal to the immune cells causing them to migrate to the area of the secretory IgA-bound particles. Imagine it this way: the bound particle acts as the dong of a dinner bell, as if to say, "Come and get it." This mechanism is well understood in respect to microbes, but few realize that it also occurs with allergic food.

Imagine what would happen if a deficiency of secretory IgA exists. Most anything would be allowed passage from the gut into the bloodstream. Unfortunately, such deficiencies are common. Nearly one-half of Americans are lacking S-IgA, while over 70% of migraine patients suffer the deficiency. This is surely one reason so many people have migraines.

It makes sense that this deficiency is common. Secretory IgA is an immune protein; therefore, anything which suppresses immune function would negatively affect it. Everything from white sugar to chlorine in the water can depress immunity. Plus, whenever a person eats an allergic food, a certain amount of S-IgA is consumed. This means that those who have hidden allergies could develop an S-IgA deficiency even if they produce adequate amounts. Intestinal overgrowth of harmful microbes known as *pathogens* greatly impairs S-IgA synthesis. Candida albicans, a yeast, is one such pathogen, and this infection is common. The pervasiveness of this infection is ultimately a result of our antibiotic era. This is because antibiotics, whether taken as a prescription or ingested through contaminated food, selectively kill bacteria, any bacteria, that exist in the body. Billions of bacteria live in a delicate ecological niche within the human intestine. Guess what happens if they are killed off, as often occurs with prescription or dietary antibiotics? Something else takes their place, and the most notorious of these is the human pathogenic yeast,

Candida. When overwhelming Candida infection occurs, the function of immune cells throughout the body becomes severely depressed and, often, the cells fail to reproduce adequately. Secretory IgA enhances natural defenses to prevent this yeast overgrowth.

Many other factors contribute to a deficiency of this important immunoglobulin. These factors may be divided into two categories, *Diseases Associated with Reduced Levels* and *Medications Reducing S-IgA Levels*, which are illustrated in Tables 1 and 2.

Table 1
Diseases Associated with Reduced Secretory IgA Levels

- Crohn's Disease
- ulcerative colitis
- celiac disease/sprue
- Addison's Disease
- ataxia-telangiectasia
- cancer
- chronic candidiasis
- chronic pulmonary infection
- amoebic dysentery
- food allergy
- giardiasis
- lupus
- irritable bowel syndrome
- peptic ulcer
- pernicious anemia
- rheumatoid arthritis
- migraine headaches
- diverticulitis

Table 2
Medications Reducing Secretory IgA Levels

- aspirin
- cortisone
- chemotherapeutic agents
- Tagament
- Clinoril
- Indocin
- antibiotics
- birth control pills
- Naprosyn
- antacids

From Table 1, it becomes clear that S-IgA deficiency is a common factor in many diseases, especially diseases of the digestive organs. Unfortunately, many individuals who have these diseases are taking medications which only further accentuate the deficiency.

How can S-IgA levels be boosted? Nutritional therapy is currently the only known way. Secretory IgA is made from protein. Therefore, adequate dietary intake is important. Certain vitamins are also needed for its synthesis. Nutrients which are useful for increasing S-IgA levels include:

- vitamin A
- vitamin B-12
- vitamin C
- folic acid
- pantothenic acid
- vitamin B-6
- cayenne pepper
- butyric acid
- thiamine
- vitamin E

One of the most valuable supplements is not a nutrient. Rather, it is bacteria, in fact several types of bacteria. These organisms are known as "good" or "beneficial" bacteria. There are several types, but the most common are *lactobacillus acidophilus* and *bifidus*. Both are normal inhabitants of the human intestines. In contrast to other bacteria, they cause no toxic or ill-effects. In fact, they enhance the production of secretory IgA.

Certain foods are rich in lactobacilli, including fermented milk products and other fermented foods such as sauerkraut. Top-quality acidophilus products which are available in the marketplace include name brands such as Prime-Life, DDS-acidophilus and Kyodophilus which is made by Wakunaga Corporation. Kyodophilus is an excellent formulation. Unlike many other products, it is stabilized against heat, and, thus, the bacteria will "hold up" if exposed to typical outdoor temperatures. It is ideal for traveling, since it requires no refrigeration (see Appendix C).

The human body has established numerous defenses against allergic reactions. Nature put her finest guardian on the front line. The measurement of secretory IgA levels in migraine patients often proves valuable. If levels are increased through natural therapies, positive results must be expected. Man is unable to ingest significant amounts of secretory IgA from foods with the exception of mother's milk and colostrum. Therefore, internal synthesis must be relied upon to fortify this critical barrier. The more that is done to increase its production, the healthier the individual will be and the more resistant he/she will become to the occurrence of migraine and other illnesses.

The Leaky Gut Syndrome: A Result of Secretory IgA Deficiency?

Many Americans have a disorder wherein their intestines are unable to prohibit the passage of bacteria, yeasts, parasites, food antigens and other large molecules from entering the bloodstream. The condition is descriptively called "The Leaky Gut Syndrome." This syndrome can be caused or aggravated by a variety of factors. Parasitic and yeast infections within the gut worsen the problem, since localized infections tend to increase the permeability of the intestines. They cause a type of inflammation within the intestinal walls which may ultimately lead to intestinal bleeding. Anemia is a common end result of parasitic infection. The point is that with all this bleeding and inflammation, there is direct access through the thin intestinal membranes to the blood. This structural pathology leads to contamination of the bloodstream by intestinal contents causing a sort of toxic waste leakage. Large, highly allergenic food molecules may pass into the bloodstream with ease. Thus, it would be no surprise that people who are afflicted with chronic parasitic or yeast infections tend to have up to twice as many food allergies as non-infected individuals.

It is almost without exception that those afflicted with Leaky Gut

Syndrome have a secretory IgA deficiency. This immunoglobulin, along with other immune defenders, helps prevent infectious organisms from gaining a foothold. Without secretory IgA, any number of noxious microbes can overgrow in the intestines. Once this occurs, they crowd out the beneficial bacteria, which only further compromises immunity and increases allergic tendencies.

As stated previously, it was once thought that the intestinal wall is impermeable to anything but the smallest molecules. In every medical school and in undergraduate biology, physiology and biochemistry classes it was taught that only the end products of digestion—amino acids, vitamins, minerals, fatty acids and sugars—could be absorbed through the gut. According to this theory, the physical barrier of the gut wall made impossible the transfer of intestinal organisms or other large molecules into the bloodstream. There was some justification to this thinking, but it should have been taught that the normal, mature intestine, free of disease, functions this way. Who has a totally normal intestine anyway?

The concept of the leaky gut was first discovered by researchers who, to their surprise, found that up to 30% of *normal humans* absorb undigested milk proteins from a single glass of milk. They also found that these symptom-free people developed measurable immune reactions to the milk proteins in the bloodstream. The reaction was called a *precipitin*, meaning that the milk protein precipitated out of solution via the phenomenon of immune complex formation.

These complexes could be deposited into the cerebral vessels, jamming up the circulation to the brain. In a migrainous female, they might end up in the uterus causing referred pain to the head and neck. The researchers also found that the more milk that was ingested, the greater the amounts of immune complexes which were found in the blood. As can be imagined, this could occur with virtually any food ranging from milk products, grains, eggs, meats, fish and poultry to fruits and vegetables.

It has been established throughout this book that incompletely digested food particles as well as certain microbes can bypass or penetrate the intestinal barrier. Even the normal intestine allows the passage of large molecules such as enzymes. The more diseased the intestines are, the more likely that the passage of harmful compounds will occur.

It is helpful to review human anatomy and physiology to understand how this occurs. The intestinal walls and the bloodstream are closely related. They have to be. It is ultimately via the circulatory system that every cell and organ is fed. Blood and lymph deliver nutrients directly to the tissues. The function of the digestive tract is to break up the food particles into a usable form. Innumerable arteries supply the digestive organs with oxygen-rich blood, and still more vessels drain wastes away from the gut. The lymphatic vessels, the "other" circulatory system, are also innumerable and are critical for assisting in the absorption of fat-soluble nutrients such as fatty acids, cholesterol and certain vitamins. Thus, the arteries, lymphatic vessels and veins serve to carry away and deliver nutrient-rich blood with its vitamins, minerals, fats and proteins.

What's most revealing is viewing how this appears at a microscopic level. The small intestine, the site where over 90% of nutrient absorption occurs, contains billions of tiny fingerlike projections called *intestinal villi*. Here is where absorption ultimately takes place. The barrier between the villi and the tiny vessels which surround it is microscopically thin. Disease, inflammation, drugs, toxic chemicals and infection all disrupt the delicate structure of the villi. The result is a leakage of unwanted substances into the circulation. A good example of the type of damage that can occur to the delicate villi is the food allergy related disease, *celiac sprue*. Also known as *gluten intolerance*, this disease leads to wholesale destruction of the intestinal villi. The entire absorptive surface of the small intestine can be obliterated—just from eating gluten-containing grains.

In gluten intolerance typically the biggest offender is wheat, although rye, oats, millet and barley also contain gluten. Gluten is the protein portion of the grain. For some unknown reason, the immune system regards gluten as a toxin and sets out to destroy it. Unfortunately, the immune warfare leads to widespread destruction of the gluten and anything near it. Since gluten has a high affinity for attaching to the intestinal villi, these villi are often the first to be destroyed. The destruction is not permanent. The intestines have an astounding ability to regenerate, and the villi are ultimately "regrown." However, the destructive cycle repeats itself every time a bit of wheat, rye, oats or barley is eaten. Anyone who reads labels knows that there is hardly a food on the supermarket shelf that is free of wheat flour, wheat germ, gluten, rye, oats, barley, malt or some other grain derivative. Designing a gluten-free diet is a major project, but the improved health that results is well worth the effort.

I am gluten intolerant. I know from personal experience that one bite of bread is enough to set the destructive cycle into motion. Wheat is the most commonly consumed of the gluten-containing grains, and there are millions of wheat addicts. Wheat products are cheap, convenient and tasty. Many people find it difficult to give up wheat. Yet, those who are gluten intolerant must do so if they wish to achieve consistently good health.

Many gluten-intolerant individuals are vulnerable to developing migraines. This is partly due to the damage that occurs within the intestines. However, a more likely mechanism is what happens when antigens of incompletely digested wheat, rye, oats or barley enter the bloodstream and are attacked by the immune system. Many of these antigens are deposited in arteries of the brain, head and neck, where massive inflammation and, therefore, pain ensue.

What can the allergy-prone individual do to protect himself/herself? The value of secretory IgA was mentioned. The body has other protective mechanisms. If noxious agents enter the bloodstream, they meet a formidable foe: the liver. Nearly all blood leaving the gut must first pass through the liver before it can enter the systemic circulation. The organ is well prepared for this. Structurally, the liver resembles a massive sieve. Nearly 1/3 of its mass is made up of specialized immune cells known as *Kuppfer cells*. These cells are essentially landlocked white blood cells. Thus, they act as a sort of "net," trapping such compounds as food antigens, bacteria and toxic chemicals. In a sense the Kuppfer cells act as a spider web-like trap for microbes. Once these microbes are trapped, the Kuppfer cells begin the final kill. Ultimately, they digest the microbes, rendering them harmless.

Every day the human liver destroys millions of microbes. One can easily imagine how the existence of a sick, malfunctioning liver could predispose an individual to all sorts of illnesses. The more overloaded the liver is with infection or inflammation, the less capable it is of preventing food antigens from gaining entry into the circulation. Liver diseases of all types make an individual more vulnerable to allergy and, therefore, migraine. A list of these diseases includes:

- cirrhosis
- hepatitis
- liver abscess
- Gilbert's disease
- Wilson's disease
- cancer
- obesity (which causes fatty liver)
- hemochromatosis (severe iron overload of the liver)
- hemosiderosis (moderate iron overload of the liver)
- Epstein-Barr syndrome

Every day the liver receives multiple doses of toxins and microbes as a consequence of what an individual eats, drinks and breathes. People with these diseases or, for that matter, any health condition should avoid contact with substances which increase liver toxicity. These include agricultural chemicals such as insecticides, herbicides and fungicides. They also include drugs, whether recreational or medical, and, of course, alcohol. Also, it would be important to avoid anything which weakens the gut wall and predisposes to the entry of microbes into the bloodstream. This is another argument against the use of aspirin for the treatment of migraines, since it weakens the stomach and intestinal walls and causes microscopic intestinal bleeding. Other medications which aggravate the Leaky Gut Syndrome and, thus, increase the likelihood of liver toxicity include:

1. Bufferin and Excedrin	8. Tanderil
2. Indocin	9. Tolectin
3. Clinoril	10. Motrin (ibuprofen)
4. Butazoladin	11. Dolobid
5. Coumadin	12. Fenoprin
6. heparin	13. Fiorinol
7. Naprosyn	14. cortisone

Anything which increases the permeability of the gut places great pressure upon the liver. Heavy drug dosages may damage the intestines to such a degree that, in a sense, the flood gates are opened. As a result, all sorts of toxic reactions due to the leakage of bowel contents are possible. Drugs can cause a serious liver disorder called *chemical hepatitis.*

Alcohol is probably the most common and certainly one of the most potent offenders. It hits the liver with a double punch; alcohol weakens the gut wall, plus it causes direct damage to the liver itself. Alcohol precipitates migraines. Nearly one half of migraine sufferers are sensitive to it. Avoiding alcohol is a must for those who wish to be cured of their migraines. Remember, one drink is enough to impair liver function in people highly sensitive to it. This sensitivity occurs especially in women. Regular consumption, i.e. one or two drinks per day, is enough to cause a certain degree of permanent liver damage in alcohol-sensitive women.

Of all alcoholic beverages, wine is the number one migraine-provoking drink, especially red wines. One reason is that wine, in addition to its alcohol content, contains several other migraine provokers. Most dominating are sulfites and tyramines. Sulfites are added as a preservative and tyramines are natural by-products of the fermentation process. Red wine can cause nasty headaches—but so can hard liquor as most any alcoholic will attest.

Food Additives: A Major Cause of Allergic Migraines

It would be admirable if the cause of migraines could be pinned down to foods and beverages alone. Unfortunately, there is another complicating factor: food additives. Food additives are defined as substances, whether natural or synthetic, which are added to original food sources. A good way to illustrate this concept is to look at an example of a natural, unprocessed food: the cucumber. One would think that a cucumber is about as natural as a food can get. However, in today's market a cucumber is no longer just a cucumber. Fresh cucumbers contain additives in the form of waxes and coatings which are added for enhancement of the visual appeal and for preservation. A pickle is worse. Pickles contain up to ten different food additives besides the garlic and dill. This is the problem with nearly all of the food supply; most of the time you just don't know what you are getting.

Sulfites: Culprit Number One

Sulfites are chemical agents supposedly used to prevent food spoilage. In reality, sulfites are utilized more to enhance the visual appeal of food than to preserve it.

It is well known that sulfites are toxic. This toxicity can be severe. The FDA has attributed several fatal allergic reactions to sulfites. Yet, this organization has failed to ban sulfites as food additives. As a result, sulfites are found in many processed foods. Just look at a few labels next time you go to the grocery store. It is common to find the words sulfite, bisulfite, metabisulfite, sodium metabisulfite, potassium metabisulfite and sulfur dioxide. Although originally a gas, sulfur dioxide, once ingested, can be metabolized to form sulfites.

All sulfite sources are potentially toxic in terms of causing both symptoms and allergic reactions. The degree of these reactions varies from person to person, but they can be severe enough to cause shock and death. This occurs rarely and only in highly susceptible individuals. Fortunately, the toxicity is usually mild, leading to illness such as flu-like syndromes, runny nose, sneezing and, of course, headache. However, a single case of death from a food additive is one too many. Our food should bring us health and vitality, not illness and premature death.

Children and adolescents are particularly vulnerable to the toxicity of sulfites. Apparently, they are less capable of detoxifying sulfites than are adults. However, adults also may be reactive, and sulfite-induced illness commonly occurs in them as well. Does all this sound serious? It does, and this is just one more reason to steer away from heavily processed, additive-laden foods.

How does sulfite toxicity occur? One way is that sulfites, once ingested, are transformed into *sulfur dioxide*. This is the same gas which is responsible for acid rain. Sulfur dioxide (SO_2) is highly toxic. It causes damage to the lungs, immune system and digestive tissues. Sulfites produce toxicity through another mechanism. It has been discovered that sulfites are easily absorbed into the bloodstream and in some instances may be absorbed immediately after ingestion. Researchers have determined that there is little or no protective barrier to impair absorption once sulfites come into contact with mucous membranes or skin. This is why they are so rapidly transported into the blood. The quick absorption places severe stress on the immune system and liver, both of which are responsible for detoxifying sulfites. If the immune system and liver are overloaded, the sulfite-sensitive individual may experience a fatal or near fatal reaction known as *anaphylactic shock*. This reaction is more likely to occur in a person already plagued with allergic problems or those with weakened immunity.

Certain nutritional deficiencies also increase the vulnerability to sulfite sensitivity. Most notable are vitamin B-12 and the mineral *moly-

bdenum. While most people are familiar with B-12, few have heard of molybdenum. This is a trace mineral naturally found in the soil and water. As a result, it is also found in wholesome foods. However, molybdenum is highly sensitive and is easily destroyed by cooking and/or food processing. For example, the refining of whole wheat grain into white flour leads to the loss of over 80% of this mineral.

It becomes easy to comprehend why molybdenum deficiency is common. What makes this mineral so important is that the key enzyme system for detoxifying sulfites is dependent upon molybdenum. In other words, without molybdenum, the enzyme becomes incapacitated. According to recent research, sulfite-sensitive individuals become more tolerant of sulfites if molybdenum is supplemented in the diet.

B-12 also assists in the detoxification of sulfites. Its value is greatest during a sulfite reaction, as supplemental B-12 has been shown to minimize the severity of the reaction. How much B-12 should be given? As much as 1000 micrograms three times daily during and for a few days after the reaction is the recommended anti-sulfite dose.

Sulfite Toxicity and Restaurant Food

Most of the publicity concerning sulfites and sulfite sensitivity has revolved around the use of these chemicals in restaurants. Here, careless or misinformed workers often add excessive amounts of sulfites to foods in an attempt to preserve visual quality and prevent oxidation. Oxidation is the process by which foods become discolored or brown. Foods which typically receive a sulfite bath include lettuce, fresh vegetables, fresh cut potatoes, fish, shrimp and fruit. Here is a rule to go by: If these foods are on a restaurant menu, they contain sulfites until proven otherwise. If there is any doubt, it is always a good idea to ask. However, many servers are unaware of how sulfites are used and have no knowledge that severe toxicity can occur. It is best to have the server ask the food preparer or the chef if sulfites were used.

A neglected area as a source of sulfites in terms of publicity is the grocery store, or maybe it should be called the "additive store." This is no play on words. Virtually every packaged food has a potentially noxious additive. Since most grocery store items are either canned, jarred or boxed, it is accurate to say that over 90% of the items in the typical grocery store contain one or more food additives capable of causing allergic reactions. Sulfites are among the most pervasive. Many are aware that dried fruits, beer and wine contain sulfites. A partial list of other foods and beverages containing sulfites includes:

- jarred fruits
- fruit drinks
- fruit salads
- tortilla chips
- soups, especially canned
- French fries and Tater Tots

- salads (deli)
- diced melon and/or
  other deli fruits
- fruit toppings and fillings
- jams and jellies
- sugar (brown or white)
- gelatin
- bakery
- pie fillings
- pop-tarts
- pancake mixes
- pancake syrup
- batters and breading
- cornstarch
- potato chips
- relishes
- pickles
- olives
- salad dressings
- potato salad
- guacamole
- gravies and sauces
- canned vegetables
- frozen vegetables (some)
- vinegars
- coffee
- instant tea
- breakfast drinks
- hard liquor
- TV dinners

Is this a list of prohibitions? It is for the sulfite-sensitive individual. If the objective is to achieve improved health, then most of these foods should be avoided.

Hundreds of drugs contain sulfites. Especially suspect are drugs which are inhaled or injected. Many oral drugs also contain sulfites. These include heart medications, steroids, antibiotics, pain medicines and muscle relaxants. There should be a public outcry over the use of sulfites in drugs and foods. They serve no useful purpose and may cause great harm.

MSG: Culprit Number Two

Like sulfites, MSG is in virtually everything. It also is heavily used in restaurants, especially oriental ones. MSG has a different usage than sulfites. It is used simply to enhance flavor and has no known nutritional value.

MSG is such a nasty compound that it really doesn't deserve to be listed in second place. It is a toxic chemical, and let it be stated so, lest anyone has a doubt.

Some researchers classify MSG as a *neurotoxin*. A neurotoxin is defined as a substance, whether natural or artificial, which exerts powerful toxicity upon the nerves and may cause permanent nerve damage. There is another dangerous side to MSG: It is a drug. So says George Schwartz, M.D., author of the provocative book, "*In Bad Taste: The MSG Syndrome.*" If you find this hard to comprehend—that a drug could be allowed to be liberally added to food—you might want to read this informative book. Turn to Page 16, where this brilliant scientist calls MSG, "a poison," and Pages 19 and 121, where he proclaims it to be a drug. According to Dr. Schwartz, MSG is found in most foods—everything from fried chicken to hamburger meat—and in a majority of packaged foods found in the supermarket. Numerous research studies on MSG are quoted in his book. Among the findings are that:

- Over twenty million Americans are highly sensitive to MSG, while nearly one third exhibit a lesser degree of sensitivity.
- Symptoms range from mild reactions to serious ones requiring hospitalization.
- If the dose is high enough, everyone will react to MSG.
- Children are highly sensitive to MSG, and chronic exposure may result in behavioral disorders or impaired intellect.
- *Brain damage* is possible if the dose is high enough and the usage is prolonged.
- MSG consumption may be associated with neurological diseases including Lou Gehrig's disease, Alzheimer's disease and Parkinsonism.

More Than Just the "Chinese Restaurant Syndrome"

Many people believe that the only way to get an MSG reaction is to eat at a Chinese restaurant which loads up its food with MSG. This is untrue. MSG is used heavily by virtually all fast food restaurants. Wherever there is breading, there is also MSG. Almost everything, in terms of fast food, is breaded these days. There are Chicken McNuggets and Kentucky Fried Chicken. There are Popeye's, Churches and Brown's fried chicken and Wendy's chicken sandwich. There are fish sandwiches, tenderloins, cheese balls, fried zucchini, onion rings and breaded mushrooms. There are veal and eggplant Parmesan, breaded pork chops, chicken fried steak and many other grease-filled and MSG-coated goodies. These *gut bombs* hit with a double punch—the toxic grease and the nerve toxin, MSG. Any experienced fast food connoisseur will be able to add a few more greasy goodies to this list.

You can get the Chinese Restaurant Syndrome at virtually any restaurant—even when entertaining in fine dining. Have you ever heard of Lawry's seasoning or Accent? Both contain as their active ingredient, MSG. They are commonly used in fine dining restaurants to flavor meats and vegetables. Thus, MSG intoxication should be renamed the "Fast Food and/or Fine Dining American Restaurant Syndrome."

There should be an additional syndrome. It is the "Grocery Store MSG Syndrome." Every supermarket in this country has foods on its shelves which collectively contain hundreds of pounds of this insidious substance. MSG has infiltrated virtually every grocery store shelf, and nearly every product contains either "MSG," "hydrolyzed vegetable protein," "autolized yeast," "hydrolyzed yeast," "vegetable powder" or "natural flavors." It's unbelievable. When you read labels at the grocery store, you discover that almost everything contains MSG. It's as if we cannot live without it. MSG has so polluted our taste buds that most people would not know what these foods taste like without it.

Isn't it sensible to presume that canned tuna, especially tuna packed in "spring water" is completely natural? It isn't, since it probably contains MSG. How about dry-roasted nuts? They are supposed to be all-natural. However, many brands are laced with MSG. What about fresh meats? Some stores add MSG to "enhance flavor." How about frozen vegetables? Those which have sauces contain MSG. It has gotten so crazy that it would be easier to make a grocery-store list of foods which do not contain MSG than a list of those which do contain it. Have a look for yourself the next time you go to the grocery store. Surely you'll find this to be true, and you'll be astonished, if not appalled, at the number and variety of foods which contain MSG.

The major difficulty in determining the presence of MSG in foods is that it can be disguised by other additive names. An extremely common one is "natural flavors." This is found in many foods, including ketchup, soups, cured meats, canned meats, noodle/pasta dishes and frozen dinners. While it cannot be stated with certainty that MSG is included as one of these natural flavors, its presence is more likely than not. This suggests that even many of the foods labeled "all natural" may not be entirely safe.

What does all this have to do with headaches? A great deal. Migraine-like headaches are one of the two most common symptoms associated with MSG sensitivity, the other being a "tight feeling around the face or neck." The MSG headache can be mild, moderate or severe. What's most problematic is that the headache often occurs days after the time of ingestion. Thus, it may be difficult to trace the cause of the headache. On the other hand, some people react almost immediately. Other symptoms associated with MSG sensitivity include:

- chest pain or pressure
- depression
- diarrhea
- dizziness
- eye pain, eye irritation or blurry vision
- fatigue
- heartburn
- hot flashes

- insomnia
- nausea
- numbness around the face
- pain radiating down the arms
- palpitations
- sore throat
- stomach cramps
- sweating
- urinary discomfort

Admittedly, it is not easy to eliminate all exposure to MSG. However, it is worth the effort to limit exposure, especially if there is a history of migraines. While some people are allergic to MSG, everyone is sensitive to it. This is because MSG is truly a toxic chemical, one that everyone should avoid.

Food Dyes: Culprit Number Three

Thanks largely to the work of Dr. Feingold, a medical doctor whose research came to light in the 1970's, many Americans have become aware that food dyes are bad for the health. Early research correlated the ingestion of artificial colorings (dyes) to children with learning disorders. A new disease called *childhood hyperactivity* cropped up about the same time. Children with this disorder were so hyperactive that they could not concentrate at school. Often they were placed in lower grades or special classes; many were drugged with Ritalin. This practice is continuing today.

What is less commonly known is that food dyes cause migraines. How these noxious compounds were ever allowed into the food supply remains an enigma. Food dyes are chemicals and toxic ones at that. Most are known carcinogens. Yet, Americans continue to consume several tons of food dyes every year. Probably the biggest culprit, in terms of migraines, is Yellow Dye #5. Ironically, its chemical structure is nearly identical to that of aspirin. In fact, it is classified chemically as an aspirin derivative, i.e., a salicylate. This means that people who are allergic to aspirin are also allergic to the dye. Another name for Yellow Dye #5 is *tartrazine*, and it may be so listed on food labels.

Yellow Dye #5 is a common ingredient in packaged or canned foods. It is found extensively in fast foods, ice cream and candies. A small list of foods or substances containing it includes:

- pickles
- relishes
- prepared salads
- canned fruit
- butter
- cheese
- margarine
- baked goods, especially those with yellow, creamy puddings
- frostings
- puddings
- hard candies
- popsicles
- ice cream
- Kool-Aid
- gelatins
- soft candies—yellow, orange or light green in color.
- colored cereals
- orange, yellow or light green fruit drinks
- Gatorade
- banana flavoring

- lime flavoring
- sherbet
- mustards (some)
- Mountain Dew
- hot dog and hamburger buns, especially those with yellowish tint
- rum
- apple and cherry turnovers
- pop tarts
- children's cereals
- wine coolers
- drugs
- multiple vitamins

Through a mechanism similar to sulfites, Yellow Dye #5 also can cause allergic shock. This usually occurs in highly allergic individuals, such as asthmatics, who are allergic to the dye. It rarely occurs in migraine patients, since their allergies result from a different mechanism. However, this does serve to point out how toxic the dye can be.

There are many other common food additives. Far more exist than can be listed. Several thousand are approved for adding into our food. The majority are synthetic chemicals devoid of nutritional value. For this reason they serve no useful purpose as far as human health is concerned. The internal chemistry of the human body—the functioning of our cells and organs—has no need for food additives. The nutritional value of a substance should be the standard upon which decisions are made concerning what is and isn't allowed into the food supply. The American public must strive to get the more toxic additives pulled off the market and out of our foods. Some of the more common food additives *known to cause allergic reactions* include:

- Nutra Sweet
- saccharin
- caffeine
- artificial flavors
- artificial colors
- caramel color
- propylene glycol
- octylgallate
- propylgallate
- carrageenan
- MSG
- sulfites
- sorbitol
- dextrin
- hydrolyzed yeast protein (contains MSG)

- shellacs and waxes
- sodium benzoate
- dextrose

Both synthetic and natural food additives can cause allergic reactions. Few of the synthetic additives have undergone careful enough scrutiny to be labeled "unequivocally safe." In a broad sense, allergic reactions are a minor concern compared to diseases such as cancer. This is serious business. Toxic chemicals do not belong in food. Some of the more well-known cancer-causing chemicals which can be legally added to food are listed below:

- coal tar derivatives (food dyes, artificial flavors)
- acetaldehyde (a nerve and brain toxin)
- propylene glycol (a component of antifreeze)
- chlorine dioxide (toxic chlorine gas, a known poison to the lungs and intestines)
- butane (lighter fluid)

This is just a small list of the many toxic chemicals which are found in our food or used in food processing. The addition of these carcinogens to food should never have been allowed. What is most puzzling is how a supposedly educated, health-conscious nation could allow such blatant negligence to occur and to continue to occur. When will we, for the sake of our personal health and that of our progeny, stand up to this crime?

Make no mistake about it, antifreeze is inedible. It is toxic even in the tiniest amount. It belongs in an automobile, not in the human body. The challenge is yours, to speak out against this madness now or wait until it is too late. Do write the food processors. Your efforts will be felt. A good example is the butter industry. They are ultra sensitive to consumer pressure. Land O' Lakes of Minnesota is now in the forefront having replaced the carcinogenic coal tar dye *Butter Yellow* with the non-toxic natural dye, *annato.* Buy Land O' Lakes butter, and let the industry know that natural is better and that going natural is the consumer preference. Believe me, the rest of the butter manufacturers and possibly the margarine producers will soon follow suit. The result will be that butter dyes made from cancer-causing substances will become a thing of the past.

Food Additives and the Migraine Patient

For the migraine sufferer, all this boils down to one concept. Processed foods, packaged foods, shelf foods and fast foods are far more likely to provoke headaches than are natural, unaltered ones. The definition of a natural food is one to which *absolutely nothing is added; no flavor enhancers, no invisible antitoxidants, no food colorings, preserva-*

tives, emulsifiers or stabilizers. Just plain, clean, fresh food—this is the safest bet.

Eating out can be a real problem for the migraineur. The reason is that there is no way to know for sure what is in the food. In most restaurants, food is heavily laced with additives. Some fine dining restaurants may be an exception. Many of these restaurants make their food from scratch, and one can more easily specify changes in the menu. Most of these restauranteurs are willing to accommodate individual health needs. Just tell them that you could have a serious allergic reaction, and watch the response. Few servers are skilled at CPR! Plus, they are scared of the liability. Isn't pain, severe pain, a serious symptom? Don't be embarrassed to take whatever steps are necessary to ensure that the things you are sensitive to are kept out of the food. Remember, you are the one paying for the service, and you will be the one to pay the price if a severe migraine strikes.

Of course, fast food restaurants are the worst of all. It would be impossible to list all the additives typically found in fast foods. Fast foods are loaded with grease, hydrogenated oils, food dyes, MSG, sulfites, artificial flavors, nitrites, sugar, corn syrup, milk, white flour, white rice, starch derivatives, Nutra Sweet, caffeine, caramel color and salt. Most of these substances can instigate headaches. The real time bomb is when several are combined at once. This "additive" effect can lead to a headache severe enough to last for days.

Despite all this, it is possible to eat out and do so safely. Any restaurant which is willing to cook fresh foods from scratch—meats, poultry, seafood, fish and vegetables—would be acceptable. In this regard, it is possible to get a meal occasionally at certain fast food restaurants. Remember one thing; it doesn't cost much more to eat at a nice restaurant. A meal at Wendy's or McDonald's can cost as much as $6.00 to $8.00, which is not much less than the price of a basic meal you can get at many supper clubs. By the time the aspirin or Tylenol is added, you just about break even.

Real Food: The Major Cause of Migraines

Up to now, the discussion has been primarily about how chemicals, toxins, synthetics, fumes and food additives can cause headaches. Could foods, by themselves, be as insidious in generating migraine headaches? They are, and in sheer numbers they cause far more migraines than do chemicals or food additives.

There are several mechanisms by which foods cause migraines. No two migraine patients are alike in terms of how they react to a given food. Plus, each person has developed his/her own specific set of food allergies. True, there are some foods which are highly likely to provoke migraines. The list usually includes coffee, wine, cocoa, tea, eggs, wheat and cheese.

While it is true that many migraine patients are allergic to these foods and beverages, a significant number are not. These patients have other food allergies equally as potent in instigating migraines. For this reason, it is difficult to make a comprehensive no-no list. There are several hundred common foods, beverages and additives. No list could be comprehensive and also be specific. Even so, the following is a list of the more common foods which, through testing and clinical experience, have been found to be common migraine provokers:

- cocoa
- coffee
- eggs
- wheat
- sulfites
- food dyes
- barley
- MSG
- cheese
- orange
- tobacco
- wine
- corn

Mechanisms of Food Allergy: Migraine Reactions

This is mentioned because the thinking in the scientific community for years has been that the protein part of the food is a major initiator of allergic reactions. Many of the aforementioned foods contain little or no protein. Yet, they commonly trigger allergic migraines. It is now known that allergic reactions can be caused by a variety of other compounds. In fact, non-protein allergic mechanisms probably cause just as many migraines, if not more, than do those initiated by proteins. Let's look at some examples.

Potatoes contain protein, but they are primarily a starchy food. A common allergic reaction to potatoes results from a contaminant found on the skin, an alkaloid produced by a fungus that grows on potato skins. Neither starch nor protein is involved. This contaminant is extremely toxic as is manifested by the severe headaches it causes.

Wine contains no measurable amount of protein. Yet, headaches resulting from drinking wine are both common and severe. Wine contains *amines*, a kind of modified amino acid (not a protein), plus sulfites, mold residues, etc. Wine, as has been previously mentioned, aggravates allergic tendencies by another mechanism: it increases the permeability of the intestinal wall, allowing easier passage of potentially toxic compounds into the bloodstream. Alcohol is a solvent. This solvent can and does cause tissue damage. The delicate tissues of the human intestines are exceptionally vulnerable to its toxic effects. In addition, people can become sensitized to the original source of their favorite drinks: grapes, in the case of wine; malt, yeast and hops, in the case of beer; and grains in the case of liquor.

Lemons and limes contain aldehydes, citrus oils and flavonoids, all of which can provoke headaches. Even the smell of a freshly cut lemon can cause a headache in certain highly sensitive individuals.

Cocoa contains *theobromines* which are chemically related to caffeine. Theobromines have direct toxicity upon the nervous system. Caffeine also operates via this mechanism.

Wheat contains a protein known as gluten. This protein, by itself, can generate migraines. It also contains highly reactive compounds known as *neuroactive peptides*. These compounds exert a direct poisonous effect upon the brain. Neuroactive peptides actually bind to brain cell membranes and prevent the absorption of a critically important compound, insulin. Without insulin the brain is unable to retrieve sufficient amounts of glucose from the blood, and the energy deprivation results in a headache.

If protein antigens do enter the blood stream, that's when the real trouble begins. All sorts of immunological and chemical reactions directed against the antigens are likely to occur. Commonly, the result is inflammation, nerve irritation, clogged circulation and reduced oxygen supply. Pain is inevitable.

These inflammatory reactions can develop locally within pain-sensitive regions of the head and neck. Or, they can occur in distant sites causing the phenomenon of referred pain. Allergy-induced inflammations within the uterus, fallopian tubes or ovaries can result in migraines during the menstrual period. Similarly, an allergy reaction that occurs within the stomach, liver or intestines can lead to head pain.

When toxic allergy reactions develop within the cranium, the result can be quite severe. Recently, researchers discovered that long-term migraine sufferers are at risk for a serious condition known as *dissecting cervical and/or cranial arteries*. This means that the arteries of the upper neck and also those within the skull may spontaneously split, leak or even burst. When an allergic migraine occurs, the arteries, especially the smaller ones, become inflamed. If this happens repeatedly over a prolonged period, scarring and other damage may result. With time, this process weakens the arterial wall.

There is an additional factor the researchers failed to consider. Most chronic migraine sufferers take heavy doses of aspirin and/or similar drugs. It is likely that this drug consumption plays an even more critical role in weakening the blood vessel walls than the allergy reactions. Nutritional deficiencies also contribute to arterial disease. Often, such deficiencies are induced by drugs. Vitamin C is critical for the formation of collagen, the protein which keeps the arteries glued together. Heavy doses of aspirin—meaning more than four aspirin per day—decimate tissue vitamin C levels. Aspirin also destroys folic acid, another nutrient needed to keep the arteries strong. It is easy to comprehend why one of the major causes of spontaneous brain hemorrhage is excessive aspirin consumption. Indocin, a drug commonly given to arthritics and gout patients, also lowers vitamin C and folic acid levels. Those taking cortisone rapidly become vitamin C and B-vitamin deficient as virtually all of the B-vitamins are wiped out by this drug. Other nutrients necessary for keeping the arteries strong which may be compromised by drug therapy include vitamin E, vitamin A, vitamin K and bioflavonoids.

Recently an astonishing medical finding was reported regarding the damaging effect of chronic migraines. Many migraine patients suffer a visual disorder: they actually lose a portion of their peripheral vision. Although the visual loss is mild, it does indicate that damage is occurring. The likely cause? Impairment of circulation to the retina due to the destruction of tiny retinal arteries and veins.

All of this is just another reminder that it is of the utmost importance to either eliminate the migraines or reduce their severity. Ideally, this should be accomplished without further compromising health with potentially toxic medications. It defeats the purpose to treat the symptoms with medicines which worsen the underlying conditions. Doing everything possible to help relieve the pain is important. Getting to the bottom of the cause and striving to cure the migraine condition is mandatory.

As a rule, allergy-induced migraines cause more pain than they do permanent damage. The impairment of lifestyle and the misery of the pain are usually the most serious things to be concerned about. Eliminating the pain usually leads to rapid and effective healing with no residual damage.

Can Food Allergies Short-Circuit the Brain?

Food allergies cause physical symptoms. Pain is one of those symptoms. Yet, could mental symptoms result from food allergies? Rarely do people directly associate eating a specific food with mental or psychological symptoms. It is now known that allergies can cause mental aberrations. Researchers have found a way, using a sophisticated neurological test, to prove that what we eat affects our brains. They actually measured toxic allergy reactions while they occurred within the brain. Let's see how this fascinating story evolved.

Decades ago researchers found that certain chemicals irritate the nervous system. Most notable of these is the pesticide DDT. It was found that the chemicals, even in very small doses, damaged the nervous system, often permanently. The brain and spinal cord were most vulnerable to this damage.

These experiments were conducted with a device known as an EMG or electromyograph. *Electro* indicates electricity, *myo* is Greek for muscle and the term *graph* is self-explanatory. Thus, an EMG is the measurement of electrical activity within muscle tissue, activity which is plotted via a graph. This test is performed by placing electrodes in the patient's muscle tissue. The muscles are stimulated using a small amount of electrical current. Under normal conditions, a certain level of activity is expected when a muscle is stimulated, and this activity is represented by the height of the spikes on the graph. When researchers exposed subjects to DDT, the height of the spikes dropped measurably. In addition, these persons developed pronounced symptoms including incoordination, weakness, slumping of posture, blurry vision, drowsiness and even the feeling of being confused or stupid. Other substances which were found to depress the EMG included perfume and cigarette smoke.

The most astounding discovery was that food—in this case the common hen's egg—could have a similar effect. A 39-year old woman was the subject of the study. Her primary problem was migraine headaches which she developed after a severe viral infection. She also complained of problems with coordination and muscular weaknesses. An EMG was performed by first testing her muscles in the normal state to get a baseline. Then she was fed two scrambled eggs. Within an hour she became ill. Her hands trembled, her speech was slurred, her posture slumped and her legs weakened. She became uncoordinated, and her muscles began twitching. At this point the EMG measured greater than a 50% reduction in muscle activity and strength. All this was due to a food allergy! Similar defects occurred after food challenges with her other migraine-provoking foods which included milk, chicken and shrimp.

Fortunately, it is unnecessary for headache sufferers to undergo such a painful ordeal as having electrodes implanted into the muscles. Yet, this does illustrate a point. Certain foods and chemicals have a direct and potent influence on brain and nerve function. All nerves arise from the brain. Nerve-related symptoms, whether painful or psychological in nature, often have a physical component. Only rarely is pain or neurological disease primarily psychological in origin. With regard to migraines, it is important to always assume that the pain is physical, not mental.

Do Children Have Migraines?

This brings us to an important subject: children. They often complain of "hurt" or pain. Children can develop headaches, even at very young ages. Allergic headaches may occur as early as 2 or 3 years of age. What is most interesting is the way they describe their headache pain. Children don't understand what constitutes a headache. All they know is that they hurt. In fact, children with migraines often fail to relate that they have head pain and may complain of seemingly unrelated symptoms such as a tummy ache. This becomes a problem, since many parents and doctors disregard the child's complaints as being largely psychological. In this regard, a common thought is that the child is complaining in order to get attention or "love."

Presumably, children have better things to do than to complain about pain. If a child says he/she is in pain, we should believe it and should try to determine the origin of the pain, making sure the pain is not due to a serious problem. We should avoid writing it off as "psychological." Believe me, most children would rather be playing in a sand box, digging holes in the ground, playing with toys, watching cartoons, making mud pies, coloring or performing some other mindless, enjoyable endeavor than they would complaining about how much they hurt. When a child says he/she has a sore throat, we listen attentively and believe. Why not pay attention when other complaints are expressed? Migraines are common in children, and they become even more common as children age. The teenage years are a time when migraines often begin, and during this time they can be quite severe. This is because the frequency of headaches due to food and chemical sensitivity increases as the immune system matures. When the immune system reaches its pinnacle of maturity, as in adulthood, the incidence of migraine also reaches its zenith.

So, when a child says he/she has pain in the head, even if at a tender, young age, do pay attention. That child may well be developing the beginnings of an allergic migraine syndrome. If this condition is caught early enough, a great deal of suffering can be aborted, not to mention problems such as aspirin, codiene and other drug dependencies.

There is a problem in diagnosing allergy-induced migraines in the very young. Their allergies change with time. Plus, blood tests are usually ineffective. It is difficult to make the diagnosis via laboratory testing, because the immune system of these youngsters is so immature that measurable reactions against foods are limited. Instead, one must attempt to establish the diagnosis through trial and error and then avoid the suspect foods. Once a child reaches age 8 or 9, accurate testing can be performed. Common headache provokers in this under-8 age group include:

- MSG
- food dyes
- salicylates
- nitrated meats such as bologna, salami and ham
- eggs
- cheese
- alcohol
- sugar
- corn
- corn syrup
- wheat
- cocoa
- milk products
- soy
- Nutra Sweet
- peanuts

It must be recognized that, for the most part, today's children have horrible eating habits. Much of their diet consists of foods which are nutritionally inadequate. Which market do the sugar-coated cereal, ice cream and candy manufacturers target? Who are the top consumers of candies, cookies, popsicles, soda, candy bars, chips and other junk foods? What group do the fast food chains target? The answer is obvious. Children get hammered and hammered hard. They are constantly eating and drinking food that should be classified as *nutritional garbage*. The consequences are disastrous. Diet-induced health problems in children are exceedingly common. The incidence of juvenile diabetes is increasing, as are diseases such as obesity, high cholesterol and cancer.

What can be done about this? A great deal, if parents take the initiative. Remember one thing. Addicted children can have one of two main reactions; they either can be worn down or hyped up by a high-sugar, junk food diet. The hyped up ones are especially tough customers to cure. This is particularly true in the early stages when attempts are first made to get them off this junk food, a stage more commonly known as *withdrawal*. That's right, these children are addicts. Whatever the efforts might be, the benefits are well worth eradicating their addictions. It is up to parents to take charge of the situation and get the kids off addictive, nutritionally depleted foods. They may well develop into pussy cats as a result and become easier to control in terms of their eating habits. The benefits can be fascinating: improved grades, better behavior, less mood swings/temper tantrums and, most important, improved health.

Believe it or not, some people actually give their children wine and/or beer to drink and think it is funny. This is far from a joke and must be regarded as a dangerous practice. Alcohol is a common cause of migraines and so are the chemicals (e.g. sulfites, preservatives, etc.) it contains. Worse, even small amounts can cause learning disorders and brain damage in youngsters. This vulnerability is partly a result of the immaturity of the nervous system. The brain cells are just beginning to develop and are growing at a very rapid rate. This means that the nervous systems of children are far more susceptible to the damaging effects of alcohol than are adults' nervous systems which are fully matured. Plus, children can become physically and psychologically addicted to alcoholic beverages much more easily during the teen or adult years if they become accustomed to "booze" early in life.

It is unlikely that people who do this to children give thought to the potentially disastrous effects down the road, but they should. They must carefully consider the implications of what they are doing: alcoholism, drug dependency, mental disorders and chronic illness are all potential results of feeding the immature some "sauce." Maybe those who do this have brain damage themselves from "pickling" their cerebral cortex with alcohol or drugs.

Alcohol can turn an adult into a child. It is an unpleasant thing to see, but it is very real. On the other hand, *alcohol in no way turns a child into an adult.* If people took heed of this, our nation would be a better place to live for all. Alcoholism leads to the destruction of everything from the home to the human body. It is a 100% minus. Even the alcohol industry is urging moderation. Let's do our best to keep alcoholism at bay by keeping alcohol out of the mouths of our babies.

White and Dangerous: Are Artificial Sweeteners Headache Promoters?

White powders have become a fixture of American culture since the turn of the century. There are hundreds of white powders. Some are chemicals, others are drugs and still others are actual foods. Cocaine is a white powder, and so is aspirin. Sugar is white. Naturally brown whole wheat flour is bleached until it becomes as white as a sheet.

White implies clean. Beautiful white linen symbolizes cleanliness and prepares us for our meal. White paper towels and tissue paper give us a clean feeling when we use them. It doesn't seem to matter how these products become white. That white toiletries, cloths and powders contain residues of bleach and dioxin, both of which are toxic, seems to make no difference. What matters is that they are white. After all, who would think of cleaning the kitchen with unbleached, environmentally safe, brown gritty-looking paper towels? We need white to be clean.

The food industry and the industrial community are aware of this mentality. They are constantly working in their labs to find new, magical white substances: enter the artificial sweeteners. Of course, these too are white powders. The other white powder, sugar, is a bit out of vogue. Even so, tons of it are still consumed daily by the American public. Much of this sugar consumption is in the form of "hidden" sugar. Ketchup, which is nearly one-third sugar, is a good example.

How does sugar become white? It is bleached with chlorine or bromine gas to form perfectly white granulated or powdered sugar. Thus, it is processed until nothing of value remains. Artificial sweeteners are not always white as a result of bleaching. They are chemical powders made synthetically in a lab, and, like many other synthetics such as drugs, they are naturally white.

Does the fact that a substance is white really mean it is safe? Cocaine is white, but it is hardly safe. So is heroin and, the ultimate in white drug refinement, crack. White does not automatically imply safety. On the contrary, any white powder must be deemed toxic until proven otherwise. Glaringly white powders or other white substances are a signal to stay away at the risk of damaging one's health. Crisco is white, and so is lard. Insecticides, herbicides and coal tar derivatives such as dioxin—all are white. So when you think of white, instead of thinking of "clean," picture a skull and crossbones! What a switch in thought that would be.

The primary artificial sweeteners available on the market are Nutra

Sweet and saccharin. Both are produced synthetically, and neither is found in nature. Both were discovered accidentally by chemists who were working on other laboratory projects. Neither has been proven safe. In fact, much evidence exists to the contrary.

An internal organ which is particularly vulnerable to the toxicity of Nutra Sweet and saccharin is the pancreas. Research has shown that both of these chemicals impair the secretion of pancreatic enzymes. Even small amounts, such as that found in a single can of pop, can measurably reduce enzyme levels. Pancreatic enzymes are of vital importance. Without them, food cannot be properly digested. The toxicity of incompletely digested food has already been discussed.

There is an additional means by which these agents cause migraines: direct chemical toxicity. This is especially true of Nutra Sweet, now a well-known cause of migraine. Nutra Sweet can act as a nerve toxin, exerting ill effects upon the brain. In fact, there are several cases on record of Nutra Sweet-induced neurological disorders, and it has caused both reversible and irreversible visual loss.

All of these effects are thought to be mediated within the brain by a highly toxic by-product of Nutra Sweet metabolism: *methanol*. This substance is also known as *wood alcohol*. Methanol, in high enough doses, causes blindness and death. No wonder Nutra Sweet consumption leads to neurological disorders and provokes migraines.

Saccharin also exerts direct toxicity to the nerves, but it is a less common cause of migraine than Nutra Sweet. One only wonders what other "sweet" white powders will be legalized for dumping into food. If the FDA won't regulate these substances more carefully, who will?

Your Fillings: Can You Be Allergic to Them?

Metal allergy does occur. Medical allergists as well as dermatologists are aware of this phenomenon. One of the most common metal allergies is to nickel, a component of metal jewelry. This allergy usually manifests itself as a skin rash at the point of contact such as under a watch or beneath a necklace. But can a person actually be allergic to his/her own fillings? It is possible, since fillings are also made of metal, but just a different type. Most people have silver fillings, or more correctly, silver-mercury fillings. There is little doubt that these fillings provoke allergy reactions and headaches.

The correct terminology for the common silver filling is *dental amalgam of the silver-mercury type*. In reality these fillings are a combination of many metals and, thus, may also contain nickel, tin, zinc and other materials. Gold fillings also contain several minerals, but these fillings are less common and rarely cause illness.

It is accurate to presume that most people, when having their cavities filled with silver-mercury amalgams, thought that the material being placed in their mouths was harmless. They had full trust in the dental profession that they would certainly have studied amalgam to be sure it was non-toxic. Unfortunately, no such thorough studies were ever performed. The fact is that over one-half the weight of these fillings consists of mercury, one of the most toxic elements known to mankind.

Mercury is best described as a *neurotoxin*, meaning it is highly toxic to the nerves. Of all nerve tissue, the brain appears to be the most susceptible. Apparently, mercury has a predilection to being deposited in the type of fat found in the brain. It simply dissolves right in. Here is a story that is significant. In the 1920's and 30's, top hats were quite popular. These hats contained an inner band that was lined with mercury. The mercury was absorbed from the bands through the facial skin and scalp into the blood and then deposited in the brain. What's most interesting is that men who consistently wore these hats were known as "mad hatters." Back then, no one had any idea why they were crazy. Now, it is known that it was the mercury that did them in.

For over 100 years that dental amalgam has been placed in teeth, everyone has been led to believe that the practice was entirely safe. Those who questioned the logic of putting mercury in the mouth were told that metal amalgams were inherently stable and that the mercury would stay in the filling forever with no chance of leaking out. As it turned out, this theory was wrong. Dental amalgams do leak mercury, and this leakage can be measured. In fact, several scientists have demonstrated that measurable amounts of mercury from dental fillings can be found in the blood, liver, kidneys and nerve tissues of individuals with silver-mercury fillings.

Who is to blame for this madness? Must the dental profession be held responsible? These are difficult questions, and there are no simple answers. However, the dental profession should be the first to issue warnings concerning the dangers of dental amalgam. Instead, they are busy "reassuring" the public that no such danger exists. They are spending millions of dollars trying to prove that amalgam is the only reliable source for quick, effective filling of cavities. If only a fraction of these dollars were spent in a positive way trying to find an alternative to amalgam, the alternative would be quickly developed, and this public menace would be eliminated once and for all. Possibly, to their surprise, they would find a public willing to make any concession if it meant less danger and better health.

The informed public wants this dangerous practice stopped. If the dental profession only knew how much was at stake, maybe they would be driven to positive action instead of wasting time making excuses.

There are several ways that amalgam provokes headaches. Being a direct neurotoxin, it weakens nerve tissue, making pain and migraine more likely. One can actually be allergic to the metals in the fillings, and this can lead to headaches. An even more powerful mechanism involves electrical currents. Metals conduct electricity. What has only recently been appreciated is that when metal is in the mouth, it conducts electricity, especially if several metals exist simultaneously. The saliva acts as the conducting medium, and the fillings act as charged poles. This electrical current is most pronounced when silver and gold fillings are found together in the mouth. It seems that this creates vulnerability to a certain type of migraine induced by biological electrical currents.

The dangers of mercury absorption into human tissues can no longer be denied. While many people are allergic to nickel or tin, nearly everyone is allergic to mercury. It is truly a universal toxin and, be assured, if it exists in the mouth, it is leaking and contaminating tissues and organs throughout the body. The best proof for this came just prior to the printing of this book. A team of researchers in Calgary, Alberta, found that dental amalgam in the typical doses to which humans are exposed, causes kidney damage. The researchers placed amalgam fillings in sheep. Shortly afterwards the sheep developed kidney damage manifested by a measurable loss of kidney function, whereas the kidneys of the control sheep remained normal. Their conclusion: Dental amalgam should be banned immediately.

There is yet another sinister effect of mercury toxicity: immune decay. Mercury destroys immune cells. These cells are responsible for absorbing any remnants of mercury found in the tissues and, thus, bear the brunt of the injury. With a weakened immunity and a damaged nervous system, it is easy to see how something as seemingly unrelated as silver/mercury fillings can be a primary cause of headaches.

I was first alerted to this connection as a medical student by a wonderful lady named Mary. She had the problem of daily or near daily migraines. Nothing seemed to help her. Megadoses of vitamins and minerals were virtually useless. Osteopathic manipulative treatments were regularly performed with only minimal relief. Acupuncture proved fruitless. Trigger point injections did little more than provide temporary relief. Finally, Mary went to a dentist knowledgeable about the problems of "modern" dental fillings. He immediately spotted the problem. Not only did Mary have silver/mercury fillings, but she had gold ones as well. The dentist felt that the two different metals resulted in the formation of an electrical current in the mouth. He was right: all metal fillings were extracted, and Mary's headaches greatly improved. Remember, nothing else touched her headaches until the fillings were removed.

Fortunately, for those who have amalgam fillings, there are hundreds of dentists throughout the country who believe in the potential toxicity of mercury and who are willing to carefully extract this poison. Dentists themselves are well aware of the dangers of mercury. When raw mercury is first mixed with other metals to form amalgam, the dentist and/or technician must handle the substance with great care. The fumes from the mercury are so toxic that they can be fatal. Special warnings on the in-office handling of mercury are issued by the American Dental Association. Masks and gloves must be worn. Yet, this noxious compound is and has been freely placed in human mouths for decades!

What can be done in the case of the migraine sufferer? Serious consideration should be given to having amalgam fillings removed. Adequate replacement fillings are available. Just be sure to search for a competent, qualified dentist who understands the problems of mercury fillings and can lead you through this, step by step.

When considering the toxicity of mercury, is it any wonder that dentists have the highest suicide rate of any profession? Is this due to stress, or is it all that mercury getting into their brains? Could the mercury be the prime cause of the depression and suicidal tendency? One study in a prominent medical journal, *The Lancet*, showed that dentists have extremely high levels of mercury in their brains and that the pituitary gland is especially hard hit. Mercury levels in the dentists' pituitary glands were up to 100 times greater than the normal. The connection to suicide becomes obvious. The pituitary controls the hormone system, and hormones control mood. A dentist with depression, agitation, anger, anxiety and suicidal ideation is probably a dentist with mercury overload of the brain.

Mercury poisoning is a serious and very real problem and, as previously mentioned, can lead to kidney damage, immune system diseases and neurological disorders. Symptoms of mercury intoxication include insomnia, memory loss, agitation, mood swings, headaches, anxiety, bleeding gums, depression, bad breath and tremors. Those who have mercury/silver fillings and are concerned about toxicity may wish to contact the Environmental Dental Association (EDA). An information packet, which includes the names and addresses of dentists practicing without the use of mercury, is available at no charge. Contact the EDA at (800) 388-8124.

Food Allergies and Migraine: Selected Case Histories

What happens in real life when a migraine sufferer has his/her allergies diagnosed and when an appropriate treatment regimen is applied? It is always nice to read about real life examples. The following pages describe several selected cases of migraine cures. The reader, if plagued with migraines, may also wish to have the opportunity to feel as good as these people now do. So read on. The cure is available for all who believe in and wish to pursue this effective approach.

Lemon allergy: the cause of horrible migraines

Miss K is a wonderful lady whose expertise is in the field of preventive health care. She fought a long-standing battle with debilitating migraines and tried everything she knew to gain relief. The migraines, occurring as often as five times per week, were severe enough to keep her bedridden and unable to work. Her work was very important to her, and she tried everything to eliminate the headaches, often resorting to consuming as many as 20 to 30 aspirin a day in an attempt to control the pain. Since she had read that allergies could be involved, she attempted to discover her allergies through the time-consuming method of food elimination—withdrawing foods and reintroducing them—as a means of determining the causative foods.

As is commonly the case with health care professionals, Miss K was resistant to the idea that she had additional hidden food allergies and that these were the likely cause of her headaches. I advised her that this was probable, but she said, "I already know what my allergies are." I insisted that she had no scientific way of knowing, and finally she relented and the Food Intolerance Test was performed. The results showed a severe citrus allergy as well as allergies to butter, pork, kidney beans, filet of sole, scallops, walnuts, apples, malt, nectarines, tobacco, cashews, coffee and mint. As it turned out, every day she squeezed a wedge of lemon into her water under the impression that this was good for digestion. While it may be a digestive aid for persons who are not allergic to it, lemon in water is a digestive disaster for those who are. Lemon contains a variety of natural chemicals which can provoke migraines. In Miss K's case, removing the lemon alone knocked out over 70% of her headaches. Most of her other headaches were caused by mint, malt, pork, coffee and tobacco. Just being in a room filled with tobacco smoke was enough to provoke an immediate headache.

Severe tobacco allergy is common and is found particularly in smokers and ex-smokers. The most likely cause of headache in smokers is the tobacco they smoke. Part of their addiction may well be a result of their tobacco allergy. Miss K, a former smoker, is now headache free, that is unless she eats one of her allergic foods or is exposed to tobacco smoke.

25 years of migraines eliminated literally overnight

Mr. D experienced headaches usually on a daily basis since 1967. Although Mr. D consulted several doctors, the cause was never determined. Sophisticated tests, including CAT and brain scans as well as an MRI, failed to determine the cause.

By the time Mr. D had arrived at my office, he had long since given up on finding any cure for his headaches. In fact, he came to see me for an entirely unrelated problem. Since his overall symptoms indicated the existence of food allergies, testing was performed. Mr. D was found to be extremely sensitive to wheat, so sensitive that a diagnosis of *celiac disease* or *gluten intolerance* was established. Gluten is the protein found in wheat and certain other grains including oats, barley, millet and rye. As described previously, wheat contains proteins called neuropeptides which are irritants to nerve and brain tissues. In people who are severely sensitive to wheat, even a tiny amount can provoke symptoms.

Mr. D had been eating whole wheat products daily for years, though he had rarely eaten white flour. He had done this because he was under the impression that "whole wheat is good for you." His perception was understandable. Unfortunately, despite the fact that whole wheat is a natural food, in his case *no wheat* is the only policy to follow. Wheat and all foods containing wheat flour, bran or germ were removed from his diet.

As wheat is in most processed foods, Mr. D's diet was rather limited. However, the extra discipline was worth it. By eliminating wheat, he also got rid of his daily headaches.

As it turned out, Mr. D was a wheat addict. He ate pasta and/or bread daily. He is not alone. There are millions of wheat addicts. For some of these addicts wheat or foods containing wheat such as cereals, crackers and bread make up over 50% of the diet. Here is a rule of thumb. Wheat addicts who have headaches are probably allergic to wheat, and wheat allergy is the likely cause of their headaches. Other foods or substances may be involved such as baker's yeast which is added to all commercial crackers, pastries, buns and breads. However, in my experience, the wheat proteins found in wheat flour, whether white or whole wheat, cause more headaches than any of the additives combined.

Migraines so severe that she pounded her head against the wall

Miss J's migraines were both frequent and intense. At times the pain was so agonizing that she pounded her head against the wall, or on a table or desk. Somehow, she insisted, this gave her temporary relief. Allergy testing revealed over 20 foods to which she was sensitive. After eliminating these foods, the headaches gradually dissipated. However, to attain more complete relief, neck injuries resulting from a car accident were treated with OMT and trigger point injections (see Chapter Six). Miss J's headaches have improved over 60%, although treatment is continuing. Her allergy profile is as follows:

scallops	cola
crab	cashews
egg	dill
molasses	sardine
corn	lobster
cheddar cheese	shrimp
soy bean	oyster
peanuts	pork
walnut	mustard
	cocoa/chocolate

Mother of two with weekly migraines allergic to all-American foods

Mrs. B's migraines were frequent and severe. Each attack lasted over 48 hours. At times they were so intense that she stayed in bed for the duration of the pain. Mrs. B's diet was heavy in the all-American staples including milk products, eggs, citrus and wheat. Oranges, orange juice and wheat bread were her favorite foods. Her allergies included the following:

egg yolk	pinto bean
pork	walnuts
butter	cashews
wheat	cottonseed oil
orange	margarine
peanuts	saccharin
kidney bean	cola
sulfites	

Mrs. B experienced a dramatic improvement in her headaches, and as long as she avoids her allergies, she is headache free. Her quality of life has improved 100%. She relates that she is happier, thinks more clearly and has more energy than she's had in years.

Any one of the aforementioned foods or substances can trigger headaches. The problem is that many commercial foods contain several of these items, and this is double trouble for headache sufferers. Take deep fried fish, for example. The fish is preserved with sulfites, and the breading contains wheat, cottonseed oil, non-fat milk and margarine. Plus, it is deep fried in more margarine, cottonseed oil and/or lard. For Mrs. B, a fried fish sandwich would amount to consuming five allergic components in the final product. A severe migraine would probably be the result.

Killer headaches due to wheat/rye allergies

Mrs. Z experienced severe migraine headaches on almost a daily basis. Often developing suddenly, the headaches were so intense as to force her to leave work. Mrs. Z was a senior receptionist in a doctor's office. Two trips to Mayo Clinic and one to the Diamond Headache Center proved fruitless. Through specialized testing, it was determined that she had a chronic yeast infection in her intestines, but, more importantly, it was found that she was highly allergic to wheat, wheat bran, rye and cheese. Removal of the allergic foods and treatment of the yeast infection led to a dramatic improvement. Mrs. Z is now headache free for the first time in 30 years, as long as she stays away from wheat and rye.

Severe secretory IgA deficiency related to migraines

Mrs. G's migraines were unusually severe. When they occurred, she became debilitated for up to three days. A week did not go by without some type of headache afflicting her. Each one was different. Sometimes they were accompanied by nausea. At other times, they were associated with visual disturbances and eye pain.

Testing determined she had a deficiency of secretory IgA. Thus, she had minimal protection against allergy reactions. Mrs. G had an allergy to limes, lemons, cocoa, butter, cheddar cheese, mozzarella cheese, nectarines, apples, English walnuts, mint and black walnuts.

Aggressive treatment was instituted which included allergy removal and nutritional therapy as a means to increase the secretory IgA levels. Currently she is much improved, although she still gets an occasional headache (about once every other month).

Sinus headache and milk products

Mrs. H. had a history of headaches which occurred primarily in the front of her face. This area is commonly known as the sinus region, and, technically, her headaches were more sinus than migraine. For over 20 years she experienced headaches which occurred as often as twice a week. Also, she complained of a long-standing problem with stuffy sinuses and post-nasal drip. However, there was another peculiar complaint: she occasionally vomited after eating, even though she had no nausea or pain. This symptom in particular was highly suspect as being food allergy in origin.

In susceptible people, food allergy reactions can lead to a phenomenon known as *pylorospasm*. The pylorus is a muscle or, to be more specific, a sphincter located where the stomach ends and the intestines begin. It controls the rate at which stomach contents are emptied into the intestines. In Mrs. H's case, allergic foods greatly irritated the nerves of the stomach which control the sphincter. The pyloric spasm was so violent that vomiting ultimately resulted. Her primary allergies were as follows:

- cocoa
- milk
- butter
- cheese
- corn
- sugar
- molasses

Mrs. H related that the vomiting commonly occurred after eating her favorite late night snack. As might be suspected, this snack contained nearly all of these substances. It was a Hershey bar and a glass of milk, a snack which often ended up in the sink. After she quit consuming this addictive snack, the vomiting and headaches disappeared. She also had relief from her sinus congestion which was likely a result of the sugar and milk allergies.

Forty-year-old realtor allergic to junk foods and sugar

Mr. W had no idea why he had migraines nearly every day. He noted that stress made them worse, so he assumed this was the primary cause. Upon inquiry, I found instead that allergies were the likely culprit. His horrible diet was loaded with junk foods, sweets and fast foods. A typical breakfast consisted of doughnuts and coffee. He frequently ate deep-fried foods such as French fries and fried chicken. Cookies and sweet rolls were his favorite snacks.

It was no surprise that Mr. W was allergic to many of the ingredients commonly found in these foods. His allergies were as follows:

- molasses
- sugar
- maple syrup
- corn
- corn syrup
- beef
- fish
- cheddar cheese
- mozzarella cheese
- yeast
- MSG
- saccharin
- margarine (cottonseed oil)

The bottom line for Mr. W was that he consumed a daily dose of most of his allergic foods. MSG is found in virtually every fast and processed food as are yeast derivatives, sugar, molasses and corn syrup. Beef and cheese are primary components of pizza, burgers and other fast foods. Margarine is used in the majority of deep frying fats. Doughnuts, sweet rolls, breads, cookies, chips and fast foods all contain margarine or other types of shortening. Mr. W's headaches disappeared within four weeks, since he strictly adhered to his new diet. This was a fantastic result for a man who thought his headaches were due to the "unavoidable" stresses of his job.

Administrator of nursing school relieved of migraines

Susan J., an R.N., had suffered with migraines for over 15 years. She tried many orthodox therapies over the years, but nothing seemed to help. She became resigned to living with the pain. After hearing me speak on the radio, she decided to investigate the allergy approach.

Susan's migraines were classical. They were usually preceded by visual disturbances and often accompanied with nausea. The nausea was most bothersome and, like the headaches, lasted for days. Susan had an unusually high pain tolerance, so she took no medicine for the headaches. As she put it, she had to tough it out, since her job was important to her. She was not about to let the pain get in her way.

Susan's primary problem turned out to be food allergy. However, she also had a severe case of chronic candidiasis secondary to antibiotic toxicity, and this illness increased the allergic tendency. Her allergies were as follows:

Severe	**Moderate**
egg	shrimp
butter	lobster
lamb	pork
tobacco	mozzarella cheese
dill seed	sugar
walnuts	molasses
sulfites	soybean
cinnamon	salicylates

Susan is now free of headache pain for the first time in 15 years. As of the printing of this book, she has yet to have a recurrence of her migraines.

Talk show host for news radio station is allergic to his own state

Jan is a respected talk show host for the #1 news radio station in Iowa. I appeared on his show numerous times. He claimed he was healthy, but it was obvious he was a mess. Like nearly every other media personality, he had horrible eating habits and constantly ate junk and fast foods. While on the air, I pressed Jan about his faulty eating habits. He did admit to having memory problems, lags in concentration and occasional bouts of fatigue especially after eating. These are cardinal symptoms of food intolerance. The pop, chip and pizza man consented to a food allergy test.

The test was performed and the results were playfully discussed on the air. As it turned out, allergy was the major problem: he had over 40 of them. They included pork, beef, butter, cheese, corn, cane sugar and cola. Jan is originally from Iowa, and, as I told him over the air, he is allergic to it! The major farm products of Iowa include corn, pork, beef and milk products.

Jan had never complained of headaches. Yet, after the allergies were diagnosed and he avoided his most addictive allergy foods, headache was the first symptom he noticed when cheating. He noted on the air that after eating a bag of corn chips, he got a "splitting headache." When he religiously avoids the allergic foods, he is headache free. Needless to say, Jan is a true believer in the migraine food allergy connection.

Took so many medications, you would expect her to rattle!

Mrs. R experienced some of the most severe migraines I have ever treated. She had all the classical symptoms: nausea, visual disturbances including loss of peripheral vision, one-sided pain, throbbing pain, etc.

Due to the severe pain, Mrs. R resorted to medication. During her 25-year battle with migraines, she popped literally thousands of pills, including aspirin, Tylenol, Advil, Sine-Aid and Excedrin. There were times when she had taken aspirin "by the handful."

Mrs. R's migraines were partly allergic and partly structural in origin. Allergy removal, manipulative treatment and trigger point therapy all were employed. The results were astounding. The frequency of headaches was reduced from five or six per week to one or less per month. Plus, when they do occur, they are far less severe and last only a few hours rather than days.

Haven't heard that laugh in years ...

Pamela, a 32-year old mother of three, experienced daily headaches. She developed headaches as a freshman in college, and they worsened with time. Toward the end of college she was diagnosed by an internist as having "migraine phenomena."

Pamela's headache pain was debilitating. She found little or no relief in medication. Doctors told her nothing could be done; she was informed that she was "high strung" and also a "worrier." These comments affected her greatly, and she began to feel "responsible" for her headaches. Guilt set in and so did depression. Yet, she always remained hopeful for a cure and stayed off addictive medicines as much as she could with the belief that one day she would conquer the headaches.

When I saw Pamela, her lifestyle was poor. Her daily headaches were of low-grade intensity, and she could count on at least one severe blasting migraine each week. Just little stresses and seemingly insignificant problems could bring on a mind-bending, throbbing bomber of a headache. It was all she could do to get the kids dressed, fed and ready for school. Then she would lie down and turn off the lights to hide from the pain. Allergy testing revealed Pamela was allergic to several foods which she commonly consumed including eggs, pork, beef, butter, cane sugar, corn, cheddar cheese, beans, asparagus and cocoa. Through a combination of osteopathic manipulative treatments, allergy elimination and trigger point injections, Pamela is now headache free. That is why her sister observed a change in her and said, "I haven't heard you laugh like that in years."

Summary

Allergies do cause migraines and so do many other things. Yet, there is little doubt that allergies to foods are the number one factor. To pursue the allergy approach is to open the door to what will likely lead to a new life, one free of pain. Take that chance if you are a migraine sufferer. It will be well worth it.

CHAPTER 5
Hormonal Disturbances:
The Number Two Cause

I t may not come as much of a surprise, at least to the chronic migraineur, that hormones are closely tied to the occurrence of migraine. Many migraine sufferers have perceived this all along. Women who have PMS migraines know that their hormonal cycles tie in closely with the headaches. Less obvious hormonal connections involve headaches which occur whenever an individual is stressed or if blood sugar levels drop. Both stress and blood sugar are largely controlled by hormones.

There are several types of hormones. Virtually all hormones are produced by specialized glands known as *endocrine glands*. In medical school we were taught about these glands in a system called *endocrinology*. A few of my colleagues went on to become specialists in this field and are known as *endocrinologists*.

Brain Cells Control Our Hormones

The ultimate power behind the hormone system is the brain. Within it are two extremely important segments, the *hypothalamus* and the *pituitary*. The pituitary is a true gland, while the hypothalamus is more or less a section of brain tissue. As the hierarchy goes, the brain or cerebral cortex—our "think tank"—controls the hypothalamus. The hypothalamus exerts direct control over the pituitary. The pituitary fully controls the rest of the hormone glands.

Our thoughts, moods and the stresses of our lives do have a direct effect through these interconnections upon the synthesis, secretion and function of hormones. Also these organs—the brain, hypothalamus and pituitary—must respond to the survival needs of the body. These are known as involuntary functions and include the rhythmic beating of the heart, breathing, blood vessel tone, digestion and nerve conduction.

The pituitary is a tiny gland about the size of a pea. However, its size in no way correlates with the importance of its function. This critical gland sends special hormonal messages to all other endocrine glands signaling when to make, or when to stop making, hormones. It also communicates to them what type of hormones to make. In this way, the pituitary controls the function of the pancreas, liver, thymus, adrenals, ovaries, testes and thyroid.

When the pituitary is overstressed, headaches can result. One way this occurs is through the phenomenon known as *hypertrophy*. The term is defined as an increase in the size of an organ secondary to excessive cell growth. This essentially means that the pituitary is swollen. People who are under emotional stress or who have faulty dietary habits are likely to develop pituitary hypertrophy.

The pituitary gland sits within the cranium in a tight space known as the *sella tursica*. Often, with migraine patients, doctors view x-rays for evidence of swollen pituitary glands which can be easily defined in this restricted region. As stated in Harrison's Textbook of Internal Medicine, *"Enlargement . . . is frequently encountered in routine skull series [x-rays] obtained in patients complaining of headaches. . ."*

The swelling places pressure on nerves in the cranium, and this causes pain. The sella tursica is a weak area in the bony structure of the skull. It does allow for some give with pressure. However, many thousands of nerve fibers are found lying on the membranes surrounding this region. The swollen pituitary may place undue pressure upon these nerves or upon the brain itself, leading to headache.

The pituitary keeps the adrenal and thyroid glands functioning properly. If these glands are weakened, the pituitary is inevitably forced to overwork which leads to the hypertrophy. Thus, it is important to cure all glandular defects in order to have a healthy pituitary and in order to prevent pituitary swelling.

People whose migraines are manifested by *pain behind the eyes* almost assuredly have swollen, overworked pituitary glands. Anatomically, the gland is very close to the eyes, and this is one reason the pain is referred there.

Besides the pituitary the most important glands involved in migraine are the adrenals and the thyroid. While the pituitary exerts control over these glands, the thyroid and adrenal glands secrete the most powerful hormones in terms of overall effects upon body functions. Sex hormone glands are also important, but their relationship to the genesis of migraine is insignificant when compared to the role played by the thyroid and adrenals.

Hypothyroidism

Hypothyroidism is defined as a measurable reduction in the function of the thyroid gland. This usually occurs to the degree that signs and symptoms occur. Migraines are one of the most common of these symptoms. Thus, hypothyroidism is a major factor to consider when evaluating patients with chronic headaches. The precise reason the thyroid is so often involved in migraine is unknown.

Hypothyroidism should be a major consideration, especially in females whose migraines occur prior to or during menses. The thyroid is involved in the metabolism of estrogens and other sex hormones. Defective thyroid function causes an imbalance in the hormone system such that symptoms including PMS, hot flashes and migraine frequently result.

These symptoms often miraculously disappear after the administration of thyroid extract. The potency and quality of the extract, which is a prescription drug, does matter. Synthetic thyroid compounds have little, if any, anti-headache effect. *Synthroid* is the name for the typical synthetic thyroid prescription. Standardized raw (all-natural) thyroid extract is more effective in blocking and/or preventing headaches. This extract is made from the thyroid glands of animals.

Women are not the only ones afflicted with hypothyroidism. It can occur in children, teenagers and adult males. In fact, it is reasonable to presume that nearly every American has a thyroid problem. Is this yet another dramatic and controversial statement? It is. Let me explain. To be more specific, anyone who has subsisted over the years on the standard American diet has an improperly functioning thyroid. For the majority, the diagnosis of hypothyroidism applies. Some have such a mild case that it is never noticed. Others have it more severely.

Why isn't this disorder diagnosed more frequently? Because in the majority of instances, blood tests will largely be negative. Yet, the hypothyroid state exists, and the signs and symptoms are there. Hundreds of doctors and many scientists are aware that hypothyroidism can occur despite normal blood studies.

It is quite a claim to state that nearly every American has a thyroid problem. Some people will find this hard to believe. Many physicians will be antagonistic to the concept. However, there is a great deal of circumstantial as well as factual evidence upon which this argument is based. Recent research indicates that at least seven million Americans have hypothyroidism to the degree that it can be diagnosed medically. The thyroid gland is among the most metabolically active of all organs. It is very sensitive to defects in nutrition. It will malfunction if even a single nutrient is deficient, let alone a whole group of them. For instance, vitamin A deficiency leads to impaired thyroid hormone synthesis as does a deficiency of zinc, copper, selenium, thiamine, vitamin B-6, vitamin B-2 or folic acid. Most Americans are deficient in these nutrients.

Malfunction, in a minority of instances, can mean aberrant or accelerated function, and this occurs in a disease known as *hyperthyroidism*. In this condition the thyroid gland essentially burns itself out. Hyperthyroidism is treated medically with powerful drugs such as radioactive iodine. However, the use of many nutritional agents such as vitamin A, natural iodine and thiamine can also help alleviate the hyperthyroid condition.

Due to its rapid rate of metabolism, the thyroid gland consumes its fair share of nutrients. Nutritional deficiencies which directly impair its function include:

- cobalt
- coenzyme Q-10
- copper
- essential fatty acids
- folic acid
- iodine
- magnesium
- niacin
- riboflavin
- selenium
- thiamine
- tyrosine
- vitamin B-6
- vitamin B-12
- vitamin C
- vitamin E

Virtually every major nutrient is needed for optimal function of this gland. Since most Americans are deficient in one or more of these nutrients, it is logical to presume that nearly everyone has a thyroid defect of some sort. While it is true that nutritional supplements stimulate thyroid function, the most important element of treatment is medication—thyroid hormone. Only doctors can prescribe this compound. Testing of thyroid function both prior to and after taking thyroid hormone is advised. However, one must be aware that the tests may all be negative, and a thyroid defect can still exist. In these instances a simple at-home test known as the *underarm temperature test* may prove useful. Otherwise, a trial of thyroid hormone followed by a re-evaluation of the symptoms may help establish the diagnosis.

As mentioned, underarm temperature can be a clue to the existence of hypothyroidism. The lower the temperature readings, the more significant are the results. This test was first developed by Broda Barnes, M.D. He found that readings consistently below 97.6 degrees Fahrenheit indicated the existence of hypothyroidism. In this instance the sluggish thyroid could no longer sustain a normal metabolic rate. The result was reduced body temperature.

Here is how this test is performed. Simply place by the bedside a standard thermometer which has been shaken down. Upon awakening, immediately place the thermometer under the arm, and don't move. Stay in bed for 10 minutes, and record the temperature. Do this for seven to ten days. Then, take an average. Women who menstruate often find that the temperature changes dramatically during this time.

What does this have to do with headaches? Migraines are common in people with hypothyroidism. Some of these individuals get headaches which never seem to go away. Patients who have continuous headaches should be thoroughly evaluated for thyroid disorders. In fact, the prolonged, endless headache is what the author describes as the *hypothyroid headache*. If the more serious causes have been ruled out, anyone who has a daily headache which lasts for weeks or months must be suspected as being hypothyroid in addition to being allergic to foods. Can it be imagined—a continuous, year-long migraine? It is possible in hypothyroidism. What is the explanation? No one knows for sure. It seems likely that the lowered body temperature and the resulting impaired metabolism make the hypothyroid individual more vulnerable to migraine attacks.

Many symptoms are associated with hypothyroidism. Thus, this condition can mimic other illnesses. To help solidify the diagnosis, a questionnaire has been devised listing signs and symptoms which are commonly found in the hypothyroid patient. Answer yes or no to the following to find out what your score is:

Hypothyroid Questionnaire

		Yes	No
1.	Do you experience constant lethargy or weakness?	☐	☐
2.	Are you tired in the morning and energetic at night?	☐	☐
3.	Do you have dry or coarse hair and/or skin?	☐	☐
4.	Is your speech slowed, or do you have slurred speech?	☐	☐
5.	Do you have swelling of the face and/or eye lids?	☐	☐
6.	Are your hands and feet cold?	☐	☐
7.	Do you experience bloating and indigestion after eating?	☐	☐
8.	Do you have hair loss from the outer third of your eyebrows?	☐	☐
9.	Do you have short-term memory loss?	☐	☐

10. Do you experience depression which is worse in the winter or on overcast days?   □   □

11. Do you have white spots on your fingernails?   □   □

12. Do you have chronic weight problems?   □   □

13. Are you easily constipated?   □   □

14. Do you experience PMS and/or menstrual disorders?   □   □

15. Do your feet or ankles swell?   □   □

16. Do your hands swell?   □   □

17. Do you have chronic headaches?   □   □

18. Are you emotionally unstable?   □   □

19. Are your nails brittle?   □   □

20. Do you exhibit lack of sweating?   □   □

21. Do you have a poor appetite or a lack of hunger?   □   □

22. Are you generally nervous?   □   □

23. Do you have pale skin?   □   □

24. Do you have a dry throat, or do you experience hoarseness?   □   □

25. Do you have hair loss (particularly females)?   □   □

26. Do you have a difficult time getting deep breaths?   □   □

27. Do you experience heart palpitations?   □   □

28. Do you have severe muscle cramps?   □   □

29. Do you bruise easily?   □   □

30. Do you have joint stiffness?   □   □

Add up the number of positive answers. If you answered up to 5 as yes, the diagnosis of hypothyroidism is possible. If you answered between 6 to 11 positively, the diagnosis is likely. If 12 to 19 were positive, the diagnosis is almost assured. Over 20 indicates a severe case of hypothyroidism.

If you have headaches and there is evidence that you are hypothyroid, rest assured of one fact: if the thyroid condition is properly treated, the headaches will improve. In fact, they may well disappear altogether. Wouldn't that be a great thing?

The Thyroid Gland and Circulation

In previous chapters it was mentioned that migraine headaches occurring over a prolonged period can lead to damage of the arteries in the head and neck. Obviously, migraine is, in part, a vascular disease.

The thyroid gland exerts significant control over the circulatory system, and this is one reason disorders of the gland are related to migraine. Thyroid hormones act directly upon the heart and are responsible for increasing its pumping ability, that is its ability to force blood through the circulatory system. Also, thyroid hormones exert powerful control over heart rate, either increasing or decreasing it.

Many years ago scientists discovered that people with hypothyroidism often have elevated cholesterol and triglyceride levels. Broda Barnes, M.D., has repeatedly demonstrated that hypothyroid patients are at increased risk for developing heart disease. The low metabolic rate and reduced carbohydrate metabolism probably account for the increased levels of blood fats, but what accounts for the higher incidence of heart attacks observed in this group? It is likely due to this fact: hypothyroid patients tend to have unhealthy arteries. The more severe the thyroid dysfunction, the worse the arteries will likely be.

Diseased arteries cause the heart to be under enormous strain. This is because arteries are supposed to be soft and flexible, making it much easier for the heart to pump blood through them. However, when the arteries harden, a condition known medically as *atherosclerosis*, the heart must pump extra hard to force blood through. Plus, the arteries supplying the heart itself can become hard, a condition known as *coronary atherosclerosis*. This further impairs cardiac function by reducing blood flow to the heart muscle itself. The term *sclerosis* indicates a scarring and hardening of the tissues often complicated by the deposition of calcium. This book is not about heart disease. Yet, the relevance to migraines is clear. Poor circulation with resultant reduced blood supply to the brain increases the risk for migraines. Plus, if the arteries of the brain are themselves diseased, the connection becomes even clearer.

There is another circulatory mechanism linking hypothyroidism to migraines. As may be recalled, the thyroid gland is regarded as the "master of metabolism." This relatively small gland controls the metabolic rate for every organ and each body function. In hypothyroidism, everything is slowed down. Another way of comprehending this is to use the term "depression." In the hypothyroid individual, every physical and mental function is depressed. Blood flow is reduced as is evidenced by symptoms such as cold hands and feet, dizziness, palpitations, etc. However, a measurable depression of cardiac function, in terms of clinical disease, only occurs in extreme cases of the disease.

A good analogy of the ill effects of decreased thyroid function is how the pistons of an engine pump when a car is started in freezing weather. The thick oil causes the pistons to move sluggishly until the entire engine warms up. With the hypothyroid individual, the engine never completely warms up. As a result, a sort of sludging of the blood occurs, and, thus, circulation to the end organs is decreased. This accounts for many of the symptoms seen in hypothyroidism, especially cold hands and feet.

Few solutions are offered to hypothyroid patients. They just keep plugging along with their sluggish disposition, depressed manner, fatigued-boring personality and, often, with their frequent headaches. They try everything to rid themselves of their health problems—some even resorting to psychiatry—but nothing provides any lasting relief.

Such patients are often given sedatives and/or mood-altering drugs including Valium or Xanax which, besides being addictive, act to further aggravate the problem by suppressing the real cause. These drugs add fuel to the fire by deepening the depression, both physical and mental. Once patients become dependent upon these agents, brain chemistry becomes altered. Then it may take weeks or months to normalize brain chemical levels. Anti-depressants and anti-anxiety medications cause a unique disease—Neurotransmitter Depletion Syndrome—another syndrome to add to the list.

Here is an important point: the brain contains its own natural anti-depressants. It has been found that medicines which numb the brain— Valium, Xanax, narcotics and the like—wreak havoc with the natural chemicals that control mood. These chemicals, known as *neurotransmitters*, include such compounds as tryptophan, serotonin, norepinephrine, acetylcholine, gamma-amino butyric acid and epinephrine.

There is another category of brain chemicals: the *endorphins*. These are the brain's natural pain killers. Endorphin levels are also depressed by medications.

It is of utmost importance to reduce or eliminate all mood-altering drugs in order to cure migraines. A list of medications which inhibit the function and/or synthesis of neurotransmitters/endorphins includes:

barbiturates
codeine
Dalmane
Demerol

Dilantin
Halcion
morphine
Restoril
Tylenol #3
Valium
Xanax

In contrast, thyroid hormones help speed up the synthesis of these important natural brain chemicals. Depression is not a sign of a drug deficiency. It is a signal that *natural* chemicals are deficient, including *thyroxine* (thyroid hormone). Giving thyroid extract is a natural way to curb depression, as well as other mood disorders, without the side effects that commonly result from taking mood-altering medications.

The Thyroid and the Immune System

The health of the immune system is closely tied to how well the thyroid gland is functioning. From reading this book, it should become clear that healthy immunity is one of the best preventions against migraines. This is because the immune cells and their secretions act as guardians, protecting the body from the harmful chemical reactions that occur as a result of food or chemical allergies. Billions of immune cells line the digestive tract, lymph tissues and blood vessels. They lie in wait for allergens and/or microbes so they can detoxify and destroy them. In addition, immune organs such as the spleen, liver, lymph nodes and thymus contain innumerable amounts of these cells.

Hypothyroid individuals exhibit impaired immunity. This is partly a consequence of the role the thyroid gland plays in controlling body temperature. Hypothyroid patients exhibit a significant, measurable reduction in body temperature. Sometimes the chill of hypothyroidism goes all the way to the bone. This can be a major problem. It is within the bone, specifically the bone marrow, that most immune cells are made. Proper synthesis of these cells is dependent upon a normal body temperature. Even a high temperature is better than a low temperature. This is what happens with a fever. A natural stimulant, fever provokes the bone marrow and immune organs to synthesize white blood cells aimed at destroying the toxin or invader. In contrast, even a slight drop in body temperature leads to reduced synthesis of white cells, often by the millions. The lower the temperature becomes, the greater the impairment is in cell synthesis. Therefore, the end result for the migraine patient will be that fewer white cells are available to combat allergy reactions. Thus, the migraines will be more frequent, prolonged and severe. Improving thyroid function helps maximize the immune response, and this may mean getting rid of the headaches—for good.

Much has been said about physical disorders of the thyroid gland. However, do the workings of the mind have an effect upon the thyroid? Prolonged emotional stress may cause thyroid impairment. In fact, stress can burn out the thyroid quicker than anything else. People who are long-term sugar addicts usually have thyroid problems, since white sugar causes thyroid burnout. Other substances which impair thyroid function include pesticides, herbicides, dioxins, solvents, hydrocarbons, heavy metals, fluoride and chlorine. Heavy metals such as lead, cadmium, mercury and aluminum bind to the enzymes needed to synthesize thyroid hormones. This is also the mechanism by which fluoride and chlorine exert their toxic effects. People who drink fluoridated water, use fluoride toothpaste or take fluoride rinses are at risk for thyroid damage.

In extreme cases, hypothyroidism can prove debilitating or even life threatening. Only a small minority develop the disease to this degree. More commonly, chronic low-level illness results. A list of diseases associated with thyroid failure includes:

- chronic candidiasis
- diabetes
- Epstein-Barr syndrome
- coronary artery disease
- atherosclerosis (hardening of the arteries)
- high blood pressure
- hypoglycemia
- intestinal parasites
- lupus
- obesity
- rheumatoid arthritis
- osteoarthritis
- Raynaud's Disease
- migraine headaches

Not every person with migraines has hypothyroidism. For those who do, major steps can be taken. In these cases it is extremely likely that, through correction of the thyroid impairment, significant improvement in the headaches will result. Overall health will be enhanced, allergies will be minimized and depression plus fatigue will largely be eliminated. These positive, comprehensive results are only to be expected by improving the function of a gland known as the Master of Metabolism.

Adrenal Insufficiency

While the thyroid gland is the master of metabolism, it is the adrenal glands that are truly the masters of all hormone glands. By themselves the adrenal glands out-produce all other endocrine glands combined in terms of total numbers of hormones. Over 45 hormones are synthesized in these small glands which are somewhat smaller than golf balls. The adrenals are found one atop each kidney.

Anatomically, the adrenal glands can be divided into two sectors. These are the *adrenal cortex* and the *adrenal medulla*. The medulla is the inside or center of the gland. Its primary function is to synthesize *adrenalin* and *noradrenalin*.

These hormones are responsible for numerous functions. Most notable is the so-called "fight or flight" reaction. Have you ever become so startled that you became "scared stiff"? Or, have you ever gotten into a heated argument to the point where you were "ready to fight"? Both of these responses are mediated by a surge of adrenalin. On the other hand, have you ever become so scared that you got a sudden burst of energy to "get the heck out," as would happen to a person being chased by a ferocious dog? This, of course, is the flight response.

Adrenalin is the agent which helps athletes become mentally prepared or "psyched up" for their competitive events. It is the chemical which flows through the blood when we are frightened by a loud noise or when we experience the fear of impending doom. Adrenalin prepares the human body for all manner of daily activities, plus some risky and unusual ones as well.

Most adrenal hormones are synthesized in the cortex which is the outer part of the gland. Cortisol, or natural cortisone, is the most dominant of these. After being produced, some hormones are stored, while a certain fixed amount is secreted directly into the bloodstream. Cortisol levels are greatest in the morning between 7:00 and 8:30.

Cortical hormones have a wide range of functions and exert significant control over the operation of the digestive, immune and nervous systems. There is hardly a single function of the human body that is not influenced by these hormones. Some of the functions/effects of cortisol include:

1) the maintenance of normal blood sugar levels

2) increased metabolism or breakdown of protein

3) increased breakdown of fats, and, in some cases, increased deposition of fats

4) suppressed white blood cell synthesis

5) suppressed immune-allergic responses

6) irritability of the nervous system

7) increased production of stomach acid

8) increased bladder pressure and urination

9) increased loss of sodium, potassium and water through the urine

People who are under stress secrete excess amounts of cortisol. It takes little imagination to comprehend the potential problems resulting from over-secretion. Excess cortisone, whether natural or synthetic, leads to suppression of the immune system to the degree that harm can be done to the internal organs. Affected organs include the stomach, intestines, liver, pancreas, spleen, thymus and kidneys.

The concept that thousands of Americans have malfunctioning, over-stressed adrenal glands was first introduced in the early 1940's by a brilliant endocrinologist, John Tintera, M.D. The validity of Dr. Tintera's work was supported and confirmed by the internationally re-nowned researcher, Hans Selye, who spent much of his life studying the negative effects of stress upon animals and humans.

What were Dr. Tintera's major findings? He determined that many of his patients suffered from a syndrome of impaired adrenal function, a condition he called *sub-clinical Addison's Disease.* In coining this syndrome, Dr. Tintera went against the established medical views of his time. As with many originators of new ideas, he was ostracized. Yet, his work survived in a book called "Hypoadrenocorticism" published by the Adrenal Metabolic Research Society. Dr. Tintera's original research and observations can be found in this book.

Tintera believed that the standard medical view of adrenal disorders was incomplete. The medical profession holds the view that the adrenal glands are involved in disease only when frank symptoms of total adrenal failure—Addison's Disease—or when symptoms of the adrenal excess, a disease known as Cushing's Syndrome, exist. No doubt, both of these diseases are serious and are often life-threatening. However, is there no in-between? Must a person always have a serious disease before a diagnosis can be made? According to Dr. Tintera, there is an in-between, and thousands of Americans have it.

If the reader has chronic, severe migraines, especially migraines which are resistant to pain medicines, it is likely that adrenal dysfunction exists. This disorder is known medically as *adrenal insufficiency* or *hypoadreno-corticism.* Both terms indicate that the adrenal glands either are no longer producing the right balance of hormones, or they are unable to produce enough cortical hormones. In other words, the adrenal glands are functioning in an insufficient fashion in respect to the number of stresses that exist in life. Pain is a stress, and the weakened adrenals are unable to cope with the elements which provoke headache pain. This also means that if migraine patients had stronger adrenal glands, it is likely that the same stimulus which normally provokes headaches no longer would.

How did the adrenal glands get in such bad shape? What could possibly have made them so weak? Why do weak adrenals cause individuals to be susceptible to pain and migraines, and why do they make a person vulnerable to allergic reactions? These questions will be answered in the following paragraphs.

Refined Carbohydrates—An Adrenal Poison?

Several things weaken the adrenal glands and lead to adrenal insufficiency. Poor diet is one of them. It might be remembered that these glands are involved in the metabolism of sugars, starches, fats and proteins; in other words, food. The role played by the adrenals in fat and protein metabolism is relatively minor in comparison to that played in carbohydrate metabolism. Carbohydrates are sugars and starches.

What greatly stresses the adrenal glands are the refined carbohydrates. The worst of these are the refined sugars—white sugar, corn syrup, maple syrup, molasses, fructose, glucose, dextrose and malt. White flour and rice are somewhat better, but not by much. Refined sugars and starches are devitalized, nutritionally deficient foods. All they do is pack a calorie load—a sugar fix, if you will. These foods place great stress on the adrenal glands, increasing the demand for the synthesis of adrenal hormones. Little, short of severe emotional stress, can slug the adrenals with a harder punch than a load of refined carbohydrates.

For most Americans, refined carbohydrates form a major part of the diet. The average consumption of sugar in the United States is a whopping 130 pounds per person per year.

Some people claim that they don't eat much sugar. It is true that certain nutritionally aware people no longer consume large quantities of sugar. However, most Americans consume excessive amounts, and if they don't currently, they probably did at one time.

Think back a little. Did you eat loads of junk food as a child, teenager or adult? Let's go all the way back. Did your mother hit the sugar or starch hard, eating such things as ice cream, candy, cookies, pastries, pop, white bread or white rice while you were still in the womb? Of course, you can't think back quite that far, but your mother knows. As an infant were you nursed on corn syrup-filled formulas, or were you given sugar water in or out of the hospital? Were you fed sugar-infested cereals for breakfast as a toddler? Or, did you receive fistloads of sugar as a small child in the form of grandma's goodies, candies, lollipops, jawbreakers, jelly beans, cookies, candy bars, doughnuts, ice cream, shakes, malts, pastries, pop-tarts, birthday cakes, caramels, taffy and gum? Did you guzzle Kool-Aid, Tang, Ovaltine, Nestle's Quik, Hershey's Chocolate Syrup in milk, chocolate milk, Hi-C, orangeade, lemonade, fruit punch or similar sugar-loaded drinks? As a toddler or teenager did you drink loads of soda pop each day or every week? Were desserts of homemade or store-bought bakery goods, pies and cakes on the daily or weekly menu? Did you junk out on sugar whenever and wherever you could?

Was white bread, white flour or pasta a staple at your home? Were crackers such as saltines, Ritz, Waverly Wafers, Wheat Thins, Cheez Nips and graham crackers common snack items? How often did you down a bunch of cookies, whether homemade or store-bought—Oreos, Hydrox, butter, oatmeal, Ginger Snaps, chocolate chip, Pinwheels, peanut butter, Pepperidge Farms or Archway? Did you often junk out on Twinkies, cup cakes, Snow Balls, Suzie-Q's, Ding Dongs, fruit pies or Little Debs? Did your gut, overall, get a constant or even intermittent blasting with these adrenal bombs? Most likely it did. There are very few exceptions, at least for anyone born since the late 1930's. The rule is, if a person lived in the USA during the 1940's through the 1990's and is under 70 years old, he/she ate enormous amounts of sugar in the form of sugar and flour-infested gut bombs, or in the form of sugar "blended into the food supply." As a result, most Americans have probably bombed out a portion of their adrenal function. In addition to the gut bombs, sugar entered the diet in more disguised forms, that is foods to which sugar is added. Cole slaw, ketchup, tartar sauce, salad dressings, bologna, hot dogs, corned beef, pork 'n beans, relish, spaghetti sauce, barbecue sauce and canned corn are just a few examples.

Are there exceptions—are there people who have lived a "sugar-free" life? They would be people who had the fortune of having highly educated, nutritionally oriented mothers and grandmothers who kept virtually all sources of refined sugar out of the house, and who monitored the diet of the children while they were at school or play. Do you know anyone who fits this description? There is another exception. It would be those individuals who naturally have huge, powerful adrenal glands able to withstand this sugar-induced adrenal stress.

If you don't fit one of these categories, then you must stay away from all gut-bombs if you wish to remain healthy, energetic and free of migraines. This is a rule that can't be broken if success is to come quickly in curing the headaches.

Several other factors besides refined sugars stress the adrenal glands. Alcohol is one of them. This is particularly true in the quantities in which it is consumed by alcoholics. Invariably, alcoholics have weak adrenals. So do smokers. Drug addicts too are giving themselves adrenal blasts. This is one reason drinkers continue drinking, smokers continue smoking and drug addicts continue shooting up. They are continually prodding their adrenals to get a temporary high. Nicotine gives smokers an adrenalin kick. However, this artificial stimulation ultimately results in a state of terrible adrenal fatigue. This is why they must continually "light up another."

Stress and the Adrenal Glands

In many illnesses, emotional and psychic stresses are the major causes of adrenal failure, playing even more of a role than diet. This kind of stress can lead to everything from weak adrenals to heart disease, heart attacks, stroke, arthritis, colitis, ulcers and cancer. Here are just a few examples of how mental stress can lead to physical damage:

1. Stress causes platelet levels in the blood to increase and also causes platelets to become more sticky. Because of this, blood clots may form more easily. Migraines are associated with an increased degree of platelet adhesiveness.

2. Medical students undertaking exams exhibit a measurable decline in immune function which increases their susceptibility to colds and flu.

3. Hans Selye found that anger causes a massive increase in the secretion of stomach acid, and that this excess acid damages the intestinal walls. He also found that anger, excitement and/or worry all place stress upon the adrenal glands, increasing the secretion of adrenal hormones.

4. Researchers known as *neuroendocrinologists* have found that stress causes the production of certain chemicals called *neurohormones*. These chemicals are very powerful and can initiate the degenerative changes that lead to many diseases including cancer, heart disease and arthritis.

Mental stress can cause illness, or it can worsen existing illnesses. To understand how adrenal stress contributes to migraines, we must return to the work of Tintera. It was stated previously that two of the major causes of migraines are allergies and low blood sugar. Adrenal insufficiency contributes to both of these. As stated by Dr. Tintera, "The chief complaints listed for patients with hypoadrenocorticism are often similar to those found in persons who are hypoglycemic." What were these suspect symptoms? They included weakness, fatigue, mood swings, headaches and faintness. Dr. Tintera found these symptoms were indeed due to fluctuations in blood sugar levels and the severity of the symptoms correlated with the lowest sugar readings. He also found that any sudden emotional upset led to further drops in blood sugar levels. Thus, when blood sugar levels were low, patients were more likely to be depressed, anxious and psychotic. Dr. Tintera quoted the work of another researcher who reported that business executives had definite drops in blood sugar levels when experiencing emotional stress.

The above data confirms that the mind affects the body. In fact, it largely controls it. As for migraine, the real problem goes back to these sudden drops in blood sugar levels which may occur several times during the day. When this happens, great stress is placed on all organs, particularly the brain. The brain uses 80% of the glucose consumed by the body. A sudden migraine attack is often the end result of this stress. When a rapid decline in blood sugar occurs, the body attempts to rectify the problem by raising blood sugar levels to normal. This is where the adrenal glands normally play an important role.

Healthy adrenal glands "kick in" by secreting the appropriate hormones to bring blood sugar levels back to normal. The weaker the adrenals are, the longer it takes for this mechanism to come into play. The result may be a prolonged battle with severe hypoglycemic migraine.

Some people believe that the answer to this type of headache would be a sugar fix. It is true that eating something high in sugar might raise blood sugar levels, but this rise would be temporary. The added stress caused by the refined sugar would further hamper adrenal function, making it that much more difficult for these glands to normalize blood sugar levels.

A possible exception to this rule is raw honey. Some headaches may actually be relieved by the consumption of large quantities of pure, unadulterated honey. What is pure honey? It is honey which has undergone minimal or no processing. Basically, this means the honey is extracted straight from the hive without undergoing excessive heating or straining. However, the honey need not be fresh, since its potency stays intact over time. Honey was found in Egyptian tombs, and it still was edible.

Patients may respond to consuming three to four ounces of pure honey several times during the day. A word of caution: honey only works for headaches due to fluctuations in blood sugar levels. Also, diabetics and severe hypoglycemics must avoid honey or any other simple sugar.

Allergy itself is a form of adrenal stress, since these glands are largely responsible for our anti-allergy coping mechanism. The connection is clear; adrenal insufficiency allows allergic reactions to proceed to an excess which leads to headaches. The severity and number of allergies is directly related to the degree of adrenal weakness. People with chronic adrenal fatigue tend to have 40 to 50 food allergies. A classic example of adrenal-induced allergy is the perfume/fume sensitivity syndrome. People who experience this are reactive to virtually any artificial and also many natural odors. Invariably, fatigued adrenals are the cause. This hypoadrenal state leads to a heightened smell sensitivity some 100,000 times normal. When the underlying adrenal disorder is treated, this chemical odor sensitivity is improved, and the allergic migraines caused by fumes will dissipate. It should also be noted that the symptoms of adrenal failure and allergy are similar. Chemical and food-sensitive individuals nearly always fit the picture of the hypoadrenal condition. The more severe the sensitivity, the weaker are the adrenals.

So many symptoms result from adrenal problems that it would be difficult to mention them all. A list of the more common ones is provided as a simple test. Take this test to see if you have adrenal problems and to also determine the severity:

Adrenal Insufficiency Exam

Do You Experience:

	Yes	No
1) constant fatigue	☐	☐
2) nervousness	☐	☐
3) irritability	☐	☐
4) depression	☐	☐
5) episodes of weakness	☐	☐
6) lightheadedness	☐	☐
7) fainting spells	☐	☐
8) headaches	☐	☐
9) heart palpitations	☐	☐
10) cravings for salt	☐	☐
11) cravings for sweets	☐	☐
12) intolerance to alcohol	☐	☐
13) intolerance to cigarette smoke	☐	☐
14) alternating diarrhea and constipation	☐	☐
15) hard, pebble-like stools	☐	☐
16) vague heartburn or indigestion	☐	☐
17) vague pains or digestive discomfort in the abdomen	☐	☐
18) food reactions/allergies	☐	☐
19) lack of appetite	☐	☐
20) infrequent urination	☐	☐

21) premenstrual symptoms □ □

22) pains in the lower neck and upper back □ □

23) pain or tightness in the upper neck or scalp □ □

24) inability to concentrate □ □

25) fears and anxiety □ □

26) periods of confusion □ □

27) impaired memory □ □

28) frustration □ □

29) compulsive behavior □ □

30) a tendency towards heat exhaustion □ □

31) cold hands and feet □ □

32) clammy, sweaty hands and/or feet □ □

33) a sense of well being after eating, especially the evening meal □ □

34) difficulty relaxing (unless working) □ □

35) excessive sweating of the palms and feet □ □

36) depression relieved by eating □ □

37) heartburn aggravated by stress □ □

38) night urination (after falling asleep) □ □

39) a tendency to have guilt feelings □ □

40) extreme sensitivity to smells □ □

41) extreme sensitivity to noises □ □

42) inability to cope with stressful events □ □

43) tendency to cry easily □ □

SCORE (as calculated by the number of questions answered yes)

0-10   This score indicates that adrenal insufficiency is likely but is probably not the primary cause of health problems. Undoubtedly, treatment of even minimal adrenal dysfunction will result in improved health, and headaches may be diminished.

11-20   Adrenal insufficiency is probably a major cause of health problems if this score applies. For treatment, a special diet low in refined sugars and starches is advised (See Dr. Igram's first book, *Eat Right or Die Young*). In addition, if the underlying adrenal disorder is resolved through nutritional and hormonal treatment, the migraine tendency will be greatly improved. Treatment also includes the use of adrenal-enhancing nutrients such as pantothenic acid, thiamine, vitamin C, vitamin A, vitamin E, vitamin B-6, Coenzyme Q-10 and carnitine.

21-30   This score indicates the existence of severe adrenal insufficiency. Such individuals usually have a history of sugar or starch addiction. A history of alcoholism and/or smoking may also be found. Treatment consists of radical changes in diet, vitamin-mineral supplementation and the addition of adrenal-enhancing herbs such as ginseng, garlic and licorice root. Daily intake of adrenal-enhancing nutrients, with emphasis on pantothenic acid and vitamin C, would also be helpful.

31-43   It is virtually definite that the diagnosis of subclinical adrenal failure applies. Medical diagnosis and treatment is advised. Treatment should be immediate in order to prevent the condition from worsening. Measures such as those mentioned above should be instituted, and special medications may be required. Of course, these must be prescribed under a doctor's care. They include thyroid hormone, natural cortisone, intravenous B-5 and B-6 and intravenous minerals such as magnesium and calcium. However, many individuals will improve dramatically once the diet is changed and appropriate nutritional supplementation is prescribed.

All this boils down to one fact. Patients with adrenal insufficiency are unable to respond positively to combat the toxicity of allergic reactions. Thus, eating the allergic food leads to symptoms. Until the immune system and adrenal glands become strong enough to cope with the allergies, symptoms will persist. Therefore, it is crucial to utilize a curative approach with the objective of rebuilding and repairing these two organs. This is so the allergic individual can cope with life and live a reasonably normal existence on this earth.

The American public is looking for safer, less invasive treatments. The medical profession must step up to the challenge and provide these alternative, non-toxic treatments.

To understand the logic behind chronic illness, all one has to do is look at the underlying physiology. Just by understanding the mechanisms of the function of the human body, things begin to make sense. Always remember the old adage coined by the father of Osteopathic Medicine, Dr. Andrew Taylor Still, who said, "Find it, fix it, then leave it be." This powerful statement summarizes the entire philosophy of osteopathy. This philosophy can be applied to migraines and virtually any other disease.

CHAPTER 6
Structural Therapies

Manipulation: A Science or an Art?

Osteopathic or chiropractic manipulative treatment (OMT/CMT) could prove to be a boon to the migraine patient. Manipulative treatment has been used for centuries as an adjunct in the treatment of illness. While there is a certain degree of science to it, OMT/CMT is primarily an art. It is a skill of the hands, of touch, of manual dexterity and of technique. It involves precision, quickness and agility. These are hardly the skills of a scientist.

It is important to understand that the quality of OMT/CMT is directly related to the skill of the operator. The strength of the operator is not nearly so important as is his/her technique. In fact, brute strength may be more of an impediment than an asset. The old adage, "The rougher the treatment, the better it feels," has no place in the art of skillful manipulative treatment.

Hopefully, this chapter will serve as a guide to the selection of a skillful manipulative therapist. There are hundreds of excellent OMT/CMT specialists throughout the country. Some of these physicians specialize in areas such as *cranial-sacral treatment,* sports medicine, low back pain, occupational injuries, etc. While few specialize in headache treatment per se, most have on record case after case of patients whose headaches improved or disappeared following manipulative treatments.

There are a few steps to take before undergoing this type of therapy. First, do some checking about the skills and reputation of the doctor before making any decision. Whether he/she has a valid medical license is not the issue. Try to determine what type of technique he/she uses and what is the practitioner's general reputation. Avoid "neck poppers," that is, practitioners who treat migraines by simply cracking the neck only. Do understand that spinal manipulation is often contraindicated *during acute migraine crisis.* In most instances, it is unwise to manipulate the neck during or right at the onset of a migraine. Often, this serves only to make the headache worse. It is preferable to wait until the headache is gone and then "straighten out" any neck lesions. Many doctors manipulate the neck during migraine attacks with good intentions and the patient's blessings. This is understandable—the pain is so agonizing that both the doctor and patient wish to attempt anything that could possibly bring relief. Yet, the severe, throbbing migraine rarely responds to this type of manipulative treatment during the migraine crisis. Some patients find more gentle techniques such as muscle-energy, soft tissue, pressure point and cranial-sacral therapy to be an exception to this rule. In contrast with acute migraines, dull low-grade tension headaches frequently can be relieved by the use of manipulative techniques, and this relief is often immediate.

There is another rule. Any time manipulative treatment causes pain, avoid it. In this instance, the definition of pain is any discomfort that lasts for days or weeks after a treatment. If necessary, seek a different practitioner who uses a more gentle technique. If pain is created as a result of the manipulative treatment, it should be mild and should disappear within 72 hours. This might be a normal result of being "realigned." This means that the muscles become sore due to assuming new postures, and the soreness should disappear within a few days. However, pain which persists despite the lapse of adequate time for healing is abnormal. Receiving further treatments would be inadvisable.

Few therapies have the attribute of being free of all side effects. Surgery has numerous side effects and so does anesthesia. Medications can cause tissue damage, sometimes permanently. Even certain vitamins can be toxic if taken in high enough doses. Some people have died from drinking too much water.

To be afraid is often to be a fool, but to proceed with caution is wise. Try not to blindly jump into anything when it comes to your health. Make sure you feel comfortable with the doctor you choose; this instinctual response is every bit as important as any investigation you might perform. Avoid doing things just to please the doctor. Try instead to please yourself.

Manipulative medicine can be good medicine. It was one of Edgar Casey's favorite remedies. He specified osteopathic manipulation. There are many good chiropractors as well. Manipulation has helped thousands with ailments ranging from arthritis to aching feet. A partial list of the conditions which may respond to skillful manipulative treatment include:

- arthritis
- asthma
- backache
- breathing disorders
- bronchitis
- bursitis
- chronic fatigue
- headache
- hip pain
- knee pain
- neck sprain or whiplash
- pinched nerve
- sacroiliac strain
- sciatica
- scoliosis
- shoulder pain
- upper back pain

Tension headache is the type that best responds to OMT/CMT. Often, the response is so beneficial that no other treatment is required. With migraines it is usually a different story. OMT/CMT acts more as an adjunctive therapy than a cure by itself. However, it is of value when combined with trigger point treatment, allergy removal and hormonal support.

Why OMT/CMT Works

Manipulation directly affects the structural components of the body. The goal is to improve the mechanical function of the joints. However, there is an additional benefit of improved structure and body mechanics. The functions of our chemistry and internal organs also improve. Structure does affect functional operations: how we breathe, how we metabolize, how we synthesize, how we circulate and how we eliminate.

Balanced structure also means more energy. This can be explained by the laws of body mechanics. It takes more energy to operate a body which has spinal lesions and joint strains than one which has none. This can be best visualized by comparing the human body to a machine. If a bearing is grinding or is stuck, it takes enormous energy to drive the machine. The machine can actually burn out its motor due to the strain. If the bearing is repaired, the mechanism runs smoothly again, and much less energy is required. A similar process occurs in the human body when a joint is "stuck." The negative effects are not quite as dramatic as would be seen in a solid metal machine, because the body is flexible and can compensate. But the loss of energy does happen, and chronic fatigue may result. If the lesion is in the right spot, there may also be headaches. If various joint strains are normalized, invariably the person will feel better, and, often, the incidence of headaches will be reduced.

Numerous structural disorders of the spine may have a negative bearing on human health and body mechanics. Many of these either cause headaches or serve to increase headache frequency and/or severity. In true fashion the tailbone is connected to the hip bone, and the hip bone to the back bone and the back bone to the neck. Just because headaches start in the head and neck, it doesn't mean this is where the major problem lies. The primary lesion might be elsewhere such as the tailbone or lower back. These regions will now be segregated for further explanation.

Neck Injuries

When it comes to migraines, injuries to the delicate structures of the neck tend to make a bad situation even worse. Car accidents are a common cause of neck injuries. Millions suffer with chronic pain as a result of whiplash-type injuries. Whiplash is known technically as *acceleration-deceleration injury.* It is so named because the neck follows the path of the impact in rear-end collisions. The neck is first jammed forward, then backward and then forward again. Tremendous forces come into play even in low speed impacts. This type of injury is extremely traumatic, and a great deal of effort is often required to normalize the tissues. The neck is highly flexible and mobile; it simply gives way and is severely twisted, strained and torqued. Frequently, the neck becomes so weak as a result of stretching of the muscles that it fatigues under the weight of the head. These symptoms may be descriptively called the Whiplash Triad: fatigue of the muscles, neck pain and headache—a combination which is often difficult to cure.

Other neck trauma may result from falls or athletic injuries. The common "pinched nerve" of the neck responds exceedingly well to manipulative treatment. Thus, headaches caused by pinched nerves are usually easily abated.

The Anatomy of the Neck

The neck can be divided into two sections: the upper part and the lower part. Strain upon the upper neck is of particular importance, since this is where the first three cervical nerves arise—C1, C2 and C3. These nerves carry the sensory fibers which are responsible for pain in the headache regions of the scalp—the posterior scalp or occiput, the temples and the frontal-sinus area. The nerves originate within the upper reaches of the spinal cord from which they exit through small canals in the second, third and fourth cervical vertebrae. Even slight strain upon the vertebrae, muscles or ligaments of this region can result in pain or make the nerves hyper-irritable. Therefore, the risk for headaches increases.

The best way to relax impinged or hypersensitive nerves is to utilize structural treatment aimed at releasing the strain. It could be massage, acupuncture, trigger point therapy, manipulation or physical therapy. However, manipulative treatment is often the quickest and easiest way to achieve results. Medications are usually worthless, since nerve impingement is a mechanical problem, not a chemical one. It requires mechanical treatment, and manipulation often works wonders—and, at times, miracles.

Mid to Upper Back

The upper and middle portion of the back have an interesting connection with headaches. This region is the site where special nerves called *sympathetic fibers* arise. Like the cervical nerves, these nerves originate within the spinal cord and exit through small canals in the vertebrae. Some of the sympathetic nerves travel directly upward into the neck and head. Others travel directly to the internal organs.

What is the importance of the sympathetic nerves in respect to headaches? They are the prime nerve system for controlling blood flow within the brain. Blood is the primary conduit for the delivery of nourishment, including oxygen. Oxygen is crucial to life. A lack of it disturbs body chemistry. Pain and inflammation usually result. The brain uses, for its weight, more oxygen than any other organ. It is ultra-sensitive to oxygen deprivation. Excessive discharge from the sympathetic nerves can cut oxygen supplies to the brain by reducing blood flow. This is because overstimulation of these nerves causes cranial blood vessels to constrict—a tightening of the tubes, so to speak. When pain-sensitive structures of the cranium are deprived of oxygen, extreme pain results. Many who have had heart or neck artery surgery are familiar with how severe this kind of pain can be. During these procedures, blood flow to the brain is actually cut off which results in severe oxygen deprivation. To watch one of these patients writhe in pain is a vivid reminder of how sensitive the brain is to reduced oxygen supply.

Researchers have proven that structural imbalance and/or trauma of the upper thoracic spine may alter the function of the sympathetics. Here again, manipulative treatment can come to the rescue and is usually the most effective method for curing structural defects.

Peripheral nerves of the head and neck are also involved in migraines. These nerves are responsible for the sensation of pain in superficial tissues which may be described as the outermost tissue layers, including the skin and the layers just under the skin.

A number of trigger points are found in the thoracic spine. When pressed, many of these will radiate a sensation directly upward toward the neck and/or scalp. For headache sufferers it is particularly important to eliminate these triggers. The triggers are often concentrated along the middle of the spine, or they may be found in significant numbers about the shoulder blade. Some headache triggers are found in such distant sites as the hands and arms. In fact, there is an important acupuncture headache point in the outer part of the hand, just up from the base of the little finger. Another one exists between the thumb and the forefinger. The complexity of the human nervous system never ceases to amaze and confound both scientists and scholars. Science has been able to comprehend only a crude, simplistic understanding of it. Even so, what is really important is what works clinically, not so much how it works. Structural therapy, including manipulation, trigger point injections and acupuncture, can knock out many of these triggers with a resultant reduction in headache pain.

The Lower Back

Lower back problems may cause or aggravate headaches. This may not come as much of a surprise. It is common for patients to say that they get a headache when their "back is out." However, few people really understand why this occurs. The lower back is vulnerable to strain and injury more so than any other region of the spine. Low back strain/sprain is one of the most common ailments occurring in America today. There are many different names for low back conditions. These include slipped disc, lumbar sprain, lumbago, pinched nerve, subluxation, sciatica, sacroiliac sprain or the more severe ruptured disc.

Whenever there is a lower back injury of any sort, it must be remembered that the lower back has a direct connection to the upper neck and the base of the skull. This connection is via a special membrane known as the *dura.* The dura is the protective membrane which encases the spinal cord. As the spinal cord ends in the lower regions of the back, so does the dura. The dura is anchored in the lower back to a region just a few inches below the lowest lumbar vertebra (L5) on a bone known as the *sacrum.* In the neck, it is tightly fixed to the 2nd and 3rd cervical vertebra. In the skull it has numerous attachments which include the occiput and all cranial bones. The occiput is the large bone in back where the neck meets the skull.

The key concept is that the dura is inelastic. It does not give, not even a fraction of an inch. Ligaments and muscles also connect the neck and skull to the lower back. However, there is a certain amount of give to these. Not so with the dura. If it is put under strain, it will pull on all of its attachments. Now the importance of these interconnections becomes clear. Strain on the lower back puts pressure on the lower attachments of the dura which pulls on the neck and head. This causes nerve tension and/or impingement, and the end result is pain.

The Tailbone

A discussion of the mechanical causes of head pain would be incomplete without including the tailbone. The tailbone is known anatomically as the *coccyx*. The dura attaches firmly here, covering most of it. Many people with chronic headaches have a history of a severe fall on the rump, such as slipping on the ice, or a fall from a height, etc. In such instances, it is possible that the headaches are partly due to a broken or dislocated tailbone. These individuals may find it difficult to sit on a hard surface and will be forced to favor one side for comfort. The person who squirms when sitting on a hard surface surely has a damaged tailbone. Other common complaints resulting from tailbone injuries include leg cramps, leg pain, difficulty taking long strides, bladder pressure, one-sided leg swelling, ankle pain and constipation.

The tailbone can be realigned through manipulative therapy. However, severe trauma can result in permanent damage. In this case, surgical correction may be necessary.

In summary, structural problems often lead to functional disturbances. This is the primary basis of the osteopathic philosophy. It should not come as a surprise that migraines or other headaches can result from structural defects. Until the mechanical/structural imbalances are corrected, it is likely that the susceptibility to pain will remain. Appropriate treatment may include quality care from an osteopathic physician, chiropractor or from a medical physician skilled in structural or manipulative treatment.

Trigger Point Injections

Nothing, short of avoiding allergic foods, has so dramatic an effect on headaches as trigger point injections. These unique injections can help relieve and/or cure migraines. They are invaluable for treating headaches caused by muscular tension. Headaches associated with *TMJ Syndrome* also may benefit. In short, trigger point injections are useful in virtually any type of headache not due to serious underlying disease.

The term "trigger point" is certainly a graphic one. That's because points of pain exist along headache regions in the scalp, temples and base of the head and neck. Many headache patients are familiar with these triggers. Often, pressing on them provides relief, although it is usually temporary. However, a true trigger is one which, when pressed, conducts a nerve sensation—a tingle of sorts—to another region. Usually, the trigger sends its impulse in a linear fashion either up or down from the point pressed. One need not press hard, since most triggers are found just under the skin. For example, a person experiencing a headache located primarily over the eye or behind the eye will often experience a shooting trigger reaction when certain occipital points are pressed. For headaches localized on the side of the head (the temple), triggers are usually found along the same side of the neck and in the scalp over the temporal region. In headaches localized to the back of the neck, triggers are almost exclusively found there in both the neck and scalp. In fact, in most types of headaches, trigger points are found in the posterior scalp and neck.

The exact nature of trigger points—what they consist of and what causes them—is unknown. Could trigger points act surreptitiously as guides for the practitioner to uncover the origin of the pain? It is sufficient to presume that they are sites of concentrated pain stimuli. This is the closest definition that can be found.

Most experts agree that, while many structures deep within the skull are sensitive to pain, headache pain arises primarily from structures outside the skull. This fact is apparent to any headache sufferer who well knows how painful the scalp, eye sockets, forehead and neck become during a headache. Pain can originate from inside the skull (*intracranially*), and, often, it feels as if this is where much of the pain comes from. Yet, researchers have found that, for the majority, headaches are caused by inflammation and irritation of pain sensitive structures such as nerves, arteries, muscle fibers, tendons and fascia located *extracranially*. Although it feels like the pain is all in the head, it is usually mostly outside the head.

The intracranial arteries, nerves and veins are sensitive to pain. However, in terms of treatment, the pain that is important is that which occurs in the superficial tissues. Most of this pain is concentrated just under the skin of the scalp, face and neck. These are the regions where most trigger points are found.

Trigger points also exist at sites seemingly unrelated to the pain such as the hands, feet, shoulders, upper back and lower back. Often, when these triggers are touched, pain radiates directly to the headache region. In some cases it is just as important to treat these distant triggers as it is to correct the local ones.

One of the most common causes of trigger points is trauma. In addition, many chronic illnesses are associated with their development. Bowel disorders, including constipation and colitis, are highly correlated. Arthritics, especially rheumatoid arthritics, tend to have numerous triggers as do individuals with sluggish metabolism such as hypothyroid patients. A list of conditions in which trigger points are commonly found includes:

osteoarthritis
rheumatoid arthritis
Epstein-Barr Syndrome
chronic hepatitis
irritable bowel syndrome
Crohn's Disease
constipation
hypothyroidism

adrenal insufficiency
migraine headaches
tension headaches
slipped or herniated disc
fibromyositis
chronic candidiasis
temporomandibular joint (TMJ) syndrome

How to Treat Trigger Points

Trigger points are localized regions of compression. They represent a concentration of forces due to factors such as muscular and ligamentous tension, vertebral displacement, injury, toxicity, edema, inflammation and nerve tension/irritability. While pressing on the trigger may provide temporary or partial relief, the quickest, most effective method of treating them is decompression. This is accomplished by "popping" the trigger via the use of injections. Popping triggers is actually quite descriptive. It is common to hear a crunching or popping noise when these regions are injected. Usually, when the pop occurs, it is associated with a sudden, measurable reduction in pain. The headache itself may not disappear immediately. Yet, sometimes it does, and there is usually a certain degree of sustained relief from the pain. More important is the fact that trigger point injections act to gradually eliminate painful stimuli which result from irritated nerves, inflamed tissues and tense muscles. By eliminating the sites of pain, one can achieve an effective, long-lasting cure in a majority of cases.

The Technique

I was first introduced to this technique by an osteopathic physician, Hal Polance, D.O., of Cedar Rapids, Iowa. As of the writing of this book, Dr. Polance has a large practice despite attempts to "slow it down."

Many of Dr. Polance's patients were headache victims whose headaches had been cured or reduced in severity via the injections. Patients would make appointments to request "the shot."

With time and experience, I modified Dr. Polance's technique. The modified technique was even more effective for eradicating headaches as well as other forms of chronic pain. It was not until I attended a medical conference in Nevada that the scientific value of this modification came to light. There, a German physician gave a lecture about the science of *Neural Therapy*. As it turned out, Neural Therapy is the German equivalent to trigger point injections. Over the years the Germans found, as I have through experience with my patients, that Neural Therapy works best if the injection is delivered immediately under the skin. The deeper the needle enters, the less pronounced is the response.

Most physicians would probably think that the needle must enter the deeper structures to deliver its medicine "on target." While this may be true of a cortisone shot into a joint, it couldn't be further from the truth when it comes to treating headache triggers. While a few injections need to be delivered at moderate depths of 1/8 of an inch or so, most should enter the skin no deeper than one millimeter. This means that the needle must be fixed just barely under the skin for the optimum effect to be achieved. Once in place, the fluid should be injected until a wheel or circle is formed. This technique is similar to that used by allergists who perform scratch testing.

Trigger points are most intensely painful during or just preceding a migraine. Often, they remain tender for a few days after the migraine subsides. Any of these situations are ideal times for trigger points to be injected.

What is injected?

The composition of the fluid that is injected depends on a number of factors. Nearly always, the principal constituent is *procaine.* Procaine is the same substance dentists use to numb teeth. It is a local anesthetic. It is commonly used by surgeons and emergency room doctors to numb injured tissue prior to suturing. A few people are allergic to local anesthetics of the *caine* family. These include procaine (novacaine), carbocaine and marcaine. Before administering the injections, it is important to ask if any known sensitivity or allergy to local anesthetics exists. If there is, other solutions devoid of local anesthetics must be utilized. The injection solution usually contains additional substances which influence nerve function and reduce cellular inflammation. These include vitamins B-12 and B-5 (pantothenic acid). B-12 by itself may be used with excellent results as can a solution of sterile salt water. What matters more than the type of fluid is where and how it is injected.

How much is injected?

Only a very tiny needle, one of the smallest made, is needed to infuse the fluid. Technically, this is a 30-gauge needle. The pain felt when the needle enters the skin is minimal. A small amount of fluid is injected, usually no more than 2/10ths of a cubic centimeter—just enough to pop the trigger point and ease the pain. Usually, multiple sites are injected in one session.

The pain from the medicine and injection is rather mild. There are many types of pain that people experience of far greater severity. There is more pain involved in having blood drawn, and a cortisone shot can't even compare. When contrasted to these, trigger point shots are a relatively painless experience.

Who can do it?

Only medically licensed physicians, D.O.'s and M.D.'s, can perform these injections. Unfortunately, only a few physicians in the United States are skilled in this technique.

Why trigger point therapy works

Dr. Harold Wolfe, a neurologist and author of the 800-page book "Headache and Other Head Pain" concluded after many years of research that, in the majority of headaches, pain arises from pain-sensitive structures located superficially. He found that pain was concentrated in the outer layers of the scalp, the skin of the upper neck, the skin around the temples, the sinuses and the superficial veins and arteries. He concluded that these tissues were ultrasensitive to pain, more so than intracranial ones. He also found the inflammation which occurred within the skull resulted in referred pain in these superficial regions. Even the deep pain which many chronic migraine sufferers experience was found to be due to irritation and inflammation of the superficial structures. Trigger point injections exert their effect on the most superficial component of headache pain.

How do painful triggers arise?

All pain arises from highly complex interactions occurring within the central nervous system. Also know as the CNS, it is divided primarily into two sections: the brain and the spinal cord. The stimulus for pain often originates from a distance, for example, from a cut or bruise. Have you ever cut yourself without knowing it only to feel pain seconds or minutes later? This is partly due to the time it takes for the injury to be evaluated and processed by the CNS. Once the CNS establishes the "need" for pain, it creates a pain reflex. This reflex is locked within the spinal cord until the need for pain disappears. This means that until a cut heals, there will be pain. Until muscle spasms ease, there will be discomfort. Unfortunately, with migraine, the pain reflex seems to become established more permanently. This pain cycle within the spinal cord remains intact until it is broken either naturally or artificially. The cycle is involuntary, but things such as mind-set, meditation, manipulative treatment, pain medicines and anti-inflammatory agents can break or diminish it. Yet, nothing seems so powerful in disrupting it as trigger point injections. Through accurate injection of triggers, the pain cycle is disengaged, often immediately. The stubborn spinal cord pain reflex seems to give up. There is usually an immediate sense of relief, as if a weight has been lifted from the head. Usually, the pain disappears within 24 to 48 hours. Ultimately, through repeated sessions, the spinal cord is tricked into losing its memory for pain, and the trigger points disappear.

Precisely why the injection of trigger points relieves local or distant pain still remains unclear. However, the technique serves as a sensible, non-toxic solution to the seemingly insurmountable problem of chronic pain. It is a safer solution than medications, but more important, trigger point therapy targets the cause, something that medications rarely, if ever, do.

CHAPTER 7
Nutrients and Migraines

Are you reading this chapter with the hope of finding a magic remedy for migraines? Unfortunately, the magic bullet for curing migraines has yet to be discovered. Neither medicine nor nutrition has developed a pill that cures this disorder. Nutrients tend to improve the migraine condition by enhancing overall health and also help increase the body's resistance to stress and pain. Hopefully, one day soon natural substances will be found which will have potent but safe drug-like pain killing powers for overcoming acute headache pain. Such a remedy may exist somewhere in Nature. It may be that we just haven't discovered it yet.

This is not to slight the value which natural compounds may have for treating migraines. Anytime overall health is improved, the resistance to illness or disease will be increased. Migraine is no exception.

There are several categories of natural compounds known to be beneficial for treating migraines. They include herbs, minerals, vitamins, amino acids, enzymes and fatty acids. Information on each of these is delineated within this chapter.

Herbs

It is unfortunate that in some circles herbs have been given a negative connotation. The use of herbs as therapeutic agents is often associated with extremism and quackery. To be sure, some herbal gurus may well practice on the fringes. Yet, to condemn herbs per se as a result of the practices of a few misguided individuals would be foolish to say the least.

Herbs are valuable for the treatment of illness, and in some instances they can cure. As many as 80% of the drugs on the market were modeled after plant and herbal derivatives. These derivatives are known as *active ingredients*. These potent ingredients are responsible for the medicinal actions of herbs.

There are thousands of herbs. It is easy to become confused by the plethora of herbs available, and still there are many thousands that are not currently on the market and thousands more yet to be discovered. Few people, except scholars in botany, have a complete understanding of the chemistry and medicinal properties of these herbs. Even the scholars have a hard time keeping up with it all.

The Chinese know a great deal about herbs. In fact in China, herbs are the main prescription for treating disease. Many Chinese medical doctors know more about herbs than they do about medications. This book will focus only on herbs for which the chemistry and mechanism of action are well understood as a result of studies reported in medical literature and which have minimal or no known toxicity.

Herbs for Migraines

Very few herbs have been studied for potential anti-migraine activity. Lately, much has been said and written about the herb *feverfew*. It has been touted as the premier natural substance for fighting migraines. It does help, but not in all cases. Plus, it is far from a cure, acting instead more like an herbal pain killer. However, feverfew is far safer than aspirin and may be worth a try. At the minimum it can be used to help reduce the dosage of the medicines. A word of caution: feverfew is botanically a weed. Therefore, allergy to it may be common. The quality of feverfew products depends entirely upon the potency of the herbal extracts and the method of their preparation (see Appendix D for recommended brands).

A favorite use of herbs and spices is a culinary one. It involves the heavy use of strong spices/herbs as flavoring agents and digestive aids. In this way, herbs and, to some degree, spices may be helpful in preventing migraines. The exception would be those who are allergic to them, and this allergy would negate any beneficial effect.

It is easy to comprehend how spices help prevent migraines. For instance, hot spices are among the top dietary sources of magnesium, the anti-migraine mineral. This infusion of magnesium into the diet can be considerable, depending upon how much and what type of spices are used. As tissue levels of magnesium rise, the propensity for migraine is decreased proportionately. In addition, hot spices are digestive stimulants. They also stimulate the metabolic rate, increasing the speed at which fats and sugars are burned as energy. Many herbs are fine sources of potassium which is an excellent nerve tonic. In addition, herbs such as ginger and turmeric contain potent anti-inflammatory compounds known as *flavonoids*. According to research, flavonoids are just as potent in reducing inflammation as many drugs.

Ginger is a case in point. It is a strong antidote for inflammations of the stomach and liver. Ginger is an effective remedy for migraines which are due to inflammation in these organs. For ginger to have a positive effect, considerable amounts must be consumed either as fresh ginger or as a supplement.

Turmeric is another valuable anti-inflammatory herb. This bright yellow substance is found in curry powder and is also used as a coloring for mustard. Turmeric can be taken in a supplemental form as a natural anti-inflammatory agent. Other herbs and spices are listed below along with the mechanism responsible for their positive effects.

Herb/Spice

hot pepper . . . . improves circulation; speeds metabolic rate

coriander . . . . one of the richest natural sources of potassium; reduces swelling

garlic . . . . improves circulation; decreases platelet aggregation

onion . . . . improves circulation; decreases platelet aggregation

licorice root . . . . reduces inflammation; enhances adrenal function

ginseng . . . . improves blood flow; enhances adrenal function

When selecting herbs and spices, choose herbs which are prepared without radiation. Unfortunately, all spices found in the grocery store have been irradiated. Do your part to boycott the use of nuclear waste to irradiate our food through buying only non-irradiated spices and herbs. These are available at fine health food stores. Hopefully, grocery stores will eventually carry them too. The more demand that is created for these quality edibles, the more likely it is that they will be made conveniently available everywhere.

Minerals

Mineral deficiency is common in migraineurs, but do minerals really provide migraine relief? To comprehend this, it is important to review the role played by minerals in human physiology.

Minerals are the stuff of life itself. Every plant is dependent upon minerals for survival. It is well known that the quality of the food supply is entirely dependent upon the health of the soil upon which it is grown, and the basis of the soil is minerals. Animals too must have minerals. In the wild they receive minerals from plants, other animals and water. Some animals even chew on rocks, coal or soil to get their minerals. Today, domesticated animals are given mineral supplements. They are fed everything from salt to selenium. Both research and the experience of farmers have determined that animals benefit from mineral-rich foods and supplements. Without minerals animals fail to thrive. Wouldn't the same be true of man?

It is likely that the reader, whether or not he/she has migraines, is mineral deficient. A person might respond by saying, "I eat a balanced diet and take a multiple vitamin/mineral supplement. I get all I need." This way of thinking is erroneous. No matter how well a person eats, mineral deficiencies still exist. Commercially grown foods are mineral deficient, often severely so. Softened water is deficient. Reverse osmosis and distilled water are totally deficient. Processed foods are super-deficient. White flour, white rice and especially white sugar are devoid of minerals. Do you know anyone whose diet is completely free of these substances? Or, do you know anyone who eats nothing but organically grown foods, foods grown on composted, mineral rich soil? How many people do you know who eat tree-ripened produce and organically raised meats? Most people have a hard time thinking of even a single person who lives this way. This is the kind of lifestyle one would have to follow to get a "balanced" amount of natural minerals.

Minerals are the spark plugs of the human engine. They act to fire-up chemical reactions. They assist in the maintenance of proper glandular and, therefore, hormone function. They help soothe and nourish the nerves and muscles.

It should be no surprise that symptoms such as fatigue, depression and anxiety are often the result of mineral deficit. One way to discover if a deficiency of minerals exists is to take the following exam:

Mineral Deficiency Exam

Which of the following applies to you?

Symptom/Condition	Deficient Mineral
1. leg cramps	Ca, Mg, K
2. toe or foot cramps	Ca, Mg, K
3. brittle or soft nails	Ca, Mg, K, Si, Fe, Zn
4. brittle bones (history of frequent fractures)	Ca, Cu, K, Si, Mn, Mg, Zn
5. history of anemia	Cu, Fe, K, Se

6.	fatigue	Cr, K, Mg, Se, Zn
7.	fall asleep after eating	Cr, K, Mg, Zn
8.	white spots on fingernails	Zn
9.	hang nails	Zn
10.	irritable nerves	Ca, K, Mg, Na
11.	high blood pressure	Ca, Cr, K, Mg, Mn, Zn
12.	ridges on fingernails	Ca, Mg, Si, Su
13.	headaches	Cr, Ca, K, Mg
14.	nerve twitching	Ca, K, Mg
15.	constipation	K, Mg, Se
16.	menstrual cramps	Ca, K, Mg
17.	kidney stones	K, Mg
18.	eczema or psoriasis	Ca, Zn
19.	impaired sense of smell	Zn
20.	elevated cholesterol or triglyceride	Cr, Mn, Se
21.	depression	Ca, Cr, K, Mg
22.	susceptible to allergy reactions	Ca, K, Se, Mo
23.	cold extremities	Ca, K, Mg, Zn
24.	hair loss or brittle hair	Cu, Si, Su, Zn
25.	anxiety	Ca, Co, K, Mg
26.	insomnia	Ca, Cr, K, Mg

KEY

Ca	..	Calcium	K	..	Potassium	Se	..	Selenium
Cr	..	Chromium	Mg	..	Magnesium	Si	..	Silicon
Co	..	Cobalt	Mn	..	Manganese	Su	..	Sulfur
Cu	..	Copper	Mo	..	Molybdenum	Zn	..	Zinc
Fe	..	Iron						

As this test demonstrates, minerals are important for the maintenance of overall health, and this function is more critical than any anti-migraine effect. Yet, certain minerals may help abort migraines, most notably calcium, magnesium and chromium.

Calcium: The Nerve Tonic Mineral

Just why calcium helps prevent migraines is unknown. However, by reviewing its functions some light can be shed on the subject. Calcium is required for normal transmission of nerve impulses. Depending upon the dose, it can act either to excite or sedate the nerves. In higher doses, it acts more like a sedative. In other words, high doses of calcium relax the nervous system. However, considerable amounts are usually needed to achieve this effect, with some 2,000 to 3,000 milligrams having been used without any known toxicity. Calcium is safe at these levels provided it is taken in divided doses throughout the day. A good anti-migraine regimen would be 750 milligrams four times daily. In severe cases during the midst of a migraine, extra doses can be taken, up to 4,000 milligrams per day. Such dosages should be taken only for a short time span. However, there is no need to worry. It is almost impossible to become calcium toxic. The body will only absorb so much. Just be sure to reduce the dose once the headache dissipates. What is a good maintenance dose? That depends upon several factors including how much calcium one is getting via the diet. In general, 2,000 milligrams per day is appropriate for anyone with chronic migraines. Women of larger frame may need 3,000 milligrams per day, while smaller-boned women might get by with as little as 1500 milligrams. It is a good idea to take a calcium supplement that contains vitamin D and magnesium, as both aid in calcium absorption. Here is the only area where caution needs to be exerted. One can get too much vitamin D. No more than 2,000 I.U. should be taken on a daily basis.

It is important to remember that most people, particularly women, lose calcium as they age. Women who smoke, drink or take the pill are especially at risk. Thus, certain women might have some catching up to do in regard to calcium intake. In addition, those who strictly avoid milk products usually have a calcium deficiency unless they are taking supplements. The prescribed dosages will give the body a chance to build up calcium levels in the bones. This ultimately means that there is more calcium available to be drawn out of the bones whenever the body needs it. The result is a calm nervous system and, thus, headaches are kept at bay.

It should be noted that many nutrients are involved in keeping the bones strong. Calcium alone is not sufficient. Also, many women are under the impression that estrogen, especially after menopause, is crucial for the maintenance of strong bones. It isn't as critical as some maintain. What is important is a balance of all the bone-building nutrients. A special multiple-nutrient formula *proven to help rebuild bone* is listed in Appendix C. Bone is a living tissue and can be renewed. Bone tissue needs a steady supply of the nutrients it thrives on. Strong bones and joints are important in headache prevention. Weight bearing is a constant stress on the skeleton and spine. The more the skeleton can withstand the pressures of gravity—jars, tumbles and mishaps of everyday life—the more resistant it will be to stress and trauma-induced headaches. Most migraine patients know that stress and structural problems can precipitate migraines. Keeping the spine strong is just one more preventive measure which can be taken.

People at extra risk for calcium deficiency headaches include:

- dialysis patients
- birth control pill users

- alcoholics
- those with a history of gastric stapling, gastric balloon or intestinal by-pass
- sugar addicts
- cigarette smokers
- coffee drinkers

Only a comparatively few foods are rich in calcium. In many of these, the calcium is difficult to absorb. For example, spinach and sesame seeds contain calcium oxalate which is poorly absorbed and can even cause some toxicity. Contrary to popular belief, calcium in milk products is relatively easy to absorb and constitutes a substantial dietary source. A recent study showed that milk calcium is absorbed as well, if not better, than typical calcium supplemental sources such as egg or oyster shell calcium. Top food sources of calcium include:

- canned salmon
- cheese (goat's or cow's milk)
- milk
- cream
- fermented milk products
- scallops
- shrimp
- herring
- sardines
- mackerel
- dark green vegetables, especially watercress, parsley and broccoli
- nuts, especially almonds

Fish are listed, because when canned, the bones are included. These bones dissolve and can be chewed. The calcium may then be absorbed. Fermented milk products are an excellent calcium source. The fermentation process makes the calcium easier to absorb. Acid assists calcium transport into the blood.

Allergy to milk products is a significant problem in migraine sufferers, and this may create difficulties in achieving adequate intake of dietary calcium. In this instance, other food sources of calcium must be regularly consumed. Watercress is one of the top vegetable sources, containing more calcium by weight than milk products. However, as with any other vegetable source, it must be well chewed or preferably juiced so that the calcium can be liberated for absorption. Carrot juice is also rich in absorbable calcium.

Magnesium: Migraine Blocking Agent?

Magnesium is the second most abundant mineral in the body. It serves several critical functions including maintenance of healthy nerves, muscles, joints and bones.

Magnesium deficiency is common and affects more than half the population. This is largely a result of the fact that the soils upon which our food is grown are magnesium deficient. It is also because processed foods contain little or no magnesium. Raw sugar pressed from the cane is rich in magnesium, but refined sugar contains none. Fresh ground whole wheat flour is an excellent source; but with white flour, some 80% of the original magnesium is lost in the refining process. The loss of this mineral in canned vegetables is over 80%, and frozen vegetables rapidly lose magnesium in the water in which they are boiled. Soft and distilled water contain no appreciable amounts. Drinking these types of water leads to magnesium deficiency. The same problem may result from drinking water treated by reverse osmosis. Mineral water rich in magnesium or purified tap water would be healthier sources.

Magnesium plays an important role as a spark plug for our cells. This spark plug action is most pronounced in the nervous system where magnesium is responsible for the initiation of nerve impulses. It is also required for contraction and relaxation of the muscles. Magnesium deficiency can lead to nerve irritability and muscular tension. In fact, when magnesium deficiency is pronounced, the muscles often become so tense that they are easily injured or torn.

Scientific evidence supports the use of magnesium in the treatment of migraines. Recent studies by doctors at the University of Tennessee showed that supplemental magnesium in a dose of 200 milligrams per day brought significant migraine relief, particularly in women. Some 80% of the women tested found their migraines to be completely gone shortly after beginning the supplements. Magnesium was so effective that it was used to stop migraines once they occurred. Many of the subjects discovered that if they took magnesium within half an hour of the migraine onset, the symptoms would abate entirely.

Migraine patients should take magnesium on a daily basis. The typical maintenance dosage would be 200 to 500 milligrams per day. An excellent, highly absorbable magnesium is manufactured by Ecological Formulas under the brand name, *Magnesium Taurate*. This type of magnesium is recommended, since it is less likely to cause digestive upset than many other brands. Magnesium is difficult to absorb. When too much magnesium enters the intestines at one time, diarrhea and cramping result. This problem appears to be eliminated by the use of magnesium taurate. Taurate stands for *taurine*, an amino acid to which the magnesium is bound. Taurine helps carry magnesium into the cells, keeping it from irritating the gut due to a lack of absorption.

Many drugs cause magnesium deficiency. A partial list includes:

- diuretics
- antibiotics
- digitalis
- aspirin
- alcohol
- calcium channel blockers
- cortisone
- laxatives

Spices, especially hot ones, and also nuts, seeds, whole grains, soybeans, dark green leafy vegetables and cocoa are rich dietary sources of magnesium. Did you see that last item—cocoa? Yes, cocoa is an excellent magnesium source, being one of the top ten sources known. Could the chocolate cravings of migraine patients be nothing more than instinctual desires to correct underlying magnesium deficiencies? It is likely, especially if these cravings occur in women around their menstrual periods, since magnesium is depleted during menses.

Chromium: Blood Sugar Regulating Mineral

Chromium is another mineral useful in the prevention of migraines. One of its most critical functions is to help drive sugar—blood glucose— into the brain. Research has shown that glucose enters brain cells up to four times more efficiently when chromium is supplemented in the diet. Our brains need extra glucose when we are under stress. Chromium may help reduce the length or severity of a migraine, especially if the migraine is due to hypoglycemia and/or emotional stress.

When people think of chromium, they often think of chrome, the metal found on car bumpers. These are two totally different things as far as the body is concerned. As can be imagined, chrome, or inorganic chromium, is very difficult to absorb. Thus, while chrome is made up of atoms of chromium, the way it exists molecularly makes absorption impossible. However, as has been borne out by numerous scientific studies, organically-bound chromium is more easily absorbed.

There are several excellent chromium supplements on the market. The names include yeast bound chromium, glucose tolerance factor, chromium picolinate and chromium nicotinate. All of these products are of value. Chromium picolinate and nicotinate are yeast free, which is important when dealing with allergic migraine. Plus, measurable, predictable responses result when these two formulations are used therapeutically. A standard dosage is 100 to 200 micrograms three times daily. Chromium picolinate or nicotinate are made by several companies (see Appendix C).

Because chromium is found in so few foods, the only reasonable way to get it is via a supplement. This is true unless one is a connoisseur of rice bran or brewer's yeast. Both of these foods suffice as chromium supplements if consumed regularly. Other good sources of chromium include organ meats, wheat germ and whole grains.

If you have migraines, be sure to build up your body levels of nerve-nourishing minerals. It may take as long as six months to replenish these levels. Taking the mentioned nutritional supplements would help, and a multiple vitamin/mineral supplement may also be necessary. However, men and post-menopausal women should avoid multiple vitamin/mineral supplements containing iron. The extra iron is not needed unless one is anemic, and it may even be harmful. Because of this, many companies offer multiple vitamin/mineral supplements which are iron free.*

Vitamins

There is no scientific evidence that vitamins relieve migraines. Most vitamins are weak in terms of anti-migraine effect. However, vitamins are important for the maintenance of overall health, and, in this regard, all vitamins are important in relation to the migraine problem. A few vitamins play an exceptional role in migraine physiology. They are pantothenic acid, vitamin B-6 (pyridoxine), vitamin C and vitamin E. By looking at the mechanism of action of these vitamins, their value in the treatment of the migraine patient is revealed.

Pantothenic Acid: Vitamin Powerhouse

Few vitamins exert as potent a biological effect as pantothenic acid. The use of pantothenic acid during a migraine may occasionally be of value, but its main use is as a tonic for the adrenal glands. This vitamin strengthens these glands and normalizes hormone synthesis. Thus, it boosts the ability of the adrenal glands to fight stress. This is the primary means by which pantothenic acid can aid the headache victim.

Regular supplementation with pantothenic acid can reduce the frequency and severity of hypoglycemia-induced headaches. Also, the adrenals will be more capable of warding off allergy reactions, reducing the likelihood of an allergy-induced migraine. Research has proven that moderate-to-high doses of pantothenic acid can induce the synthesis of adrenal steroids. These extra steroids help prevent allergy reactions, reduce inflammation and keep blood sugar levels stable. As stated previously, weakened or over-stressed adrenals are unable to keep the blood sugar on an even keel. Thus, even a seemingly slight stress such as forget-

---

* The subject of iron toxicity is discussed in detail in Dr. Igram's first book, *Eat Right or Die Young*, which is available by request at many book and health food stores, or by mail order (319) 366-5335.

ting breakfast, the aggravation of being stuck in traffic or a few whiffs of roadway fumes can bring on a headache. Remember the brain must have its glucose fix, since glucose is the only readily available source for the brain's food. A sudden drop in blood sugar levels often affects the brain, and this is manifested by mental symptoms. Here is where pantothenic acid plays one of its most critical roles. It can induce a rapid increase in the production and secretion of adrenal hormones. Once these hormones enter the bloodstream, blood sugar levels are normalized.

The recommended dosage may vary depending upon the severity of stress or the headache history. A typical maintenance dose would be 500 milligrams three times daily. This should be taken in conjunction with B-complex supplements, as the B-vitamins work best if all are available to the tissues at the same time. Up to three grams can be taken daily with no known toxicity. However, there is one negative result from taking such high doses: the inside of the nose can become dry. If you notice this, it would be wise to reduce the dose although there is no long-term ill effects of this dryness.

Excellent pantothenic acid supplements are made by several companies. Some of these companies make time-released products. In the case of pantothenic acid, time-released is good, since this vitamin can be absorbed throughout the intestinal tract. This is not true of many other B-vitamins. Another excellent formulation is made by Cardiovascular Research and is called Pantothene. This is a special form of pantothenic acid. Pantothene is of exceptional value, since it can be taken in high doses with less risk of toxicity. This is important during a migraine crisis when high doses of pantothenic acid may be useful. In addition, studies show that supplementation with Pantothene leads to improved circulation by inhibiting platelet adherence, a phenomena which contributes to migraine pathology.

Vitamin B-6: Nature's Diuretic

Vitamin B-6 is an important migraine prevention agent. This vitamin has a natural diuretic action, stimulating the kidneys to excrete excess water. Allergy reactions cause water retention and can even lead to the accumulation of water in the brain. B-6 exerts its diuretic action most profoundly when combined with essential fatty acids such as GLA or flaxseed oil.

B-6 is involved in other important functions relative to migraine. These involve the synthesis of brain chemicals known as *neurotransmitters*. Along with magnesium, B-6 is required for the synthesis and function of these neurological chemicals. Care must be taken in "megadose" B-6 therapy, since it could lead to toxicity. An excellent, non-toxic form of B-6 is available. It is called *P-5-P* which stands for *pyridoxal-5-phosphate*. A way to avoid B-6 toxicity is to take 50 to 100 milligrams of

P-5-P whenever taking more than 100 milligrams of regular B-6. By doing this, higher doses can be taken with safety. However, such dosages should not exceed 500 milligrams per day. The exceptions are certain rare diseases involving genetic defects.

Vitamin C: The Natural Antihistamine

Vitamin C is a powerhouse vitamin. It helps prevent allergic reactions by boosting immune defenses. It strengthens the adrenal glands and is required for the synthesis of all adrenal hormones. Vitamin C is Nature's antihistamine. With all these functions, vitamin C helps block the allergic reactions which lead to migraines.

Histamine is a major player in allergic reactions. It is a natural chemical which is released in large quantities from certain types of white blood cells, known as mast cells, as a consequence of allergic reactions. Migraine headaches, being primarily allergic in origin, are associated with increased histamine levels. Histamine itself, if injected into the body, can provoke migraines in susceptible individuals. For these reasons, it is important to prevent histamine levels from rising. Vitamin C, in doses of 2 to 6 grams daily, can be helpful in blocking histamine release.

Vitamin E: Blood Flow Performer

For years it has been known that vitamin E exerts many of its beneficial effects by improving blood flow. However, there is little evidence that vitamin E relieves migraines. Vitamin E does increase the ability of the blood to carry oxygen. It acts as a natural blood thinner and improves the ability of the heart to pump blood. Vitamin E also upgrades the immune response and is an anti-inflammatory agent.

Even though it is fat soluble, vitamin E is one of the safest vitamins known and can be taken in high doses without toxicity. There is one exception. Certain people with high blood pressure must proceed with caution when taking vitamin E. Blood pressure may be raised with dosages higher than 400 I.U. However, in most instances, taking vitamin E during a headache will do more good than harm.

Some people who are allergic to soy are worried that they might be allergic to vitamin E made from soy oil. This can be a problem, but most soy allergies are to soy protein. Vitamin E comes from the oil. However, wheat germ oil is used in some vitamin E preparations, and wheat-sensitive individuals need to avoid such products. Previous experiences with patients has proven that wheat allergic individuals can get a migraine from consuming wheat germ oil or vitamin E products containing it.*

Other vitamins are important. They include vitamin C, thiamine, ri-

* A vitamin E product is available which contains no added soy or wheat germ oil (See Appendix C).

boflavin, niacin, biotin and folic acid. It would be wise to take a multiple vitamin supplement containing all of these nutrients.

Amino Acids

When most people think of nutrients, they think primarily of vitamins and minerals. This is understandable. It has been taught that vitamins and minerals are essential and that we must get them via the diet to remain healthy. However, there is another group of essential nutrients: the amino acids.

Over 30 amino acids exist, although only eight are classified as "essential." By definition, essential means that the nutrient cannot be made within the human body and, therefore, must be obtained via dietary sources. For example, our bodies cannot synthesize calcium, nor can they make the amino acid *phenlyalanine*. Some vitamins can be synthesized, but the majority are essential, since they must be received through the diet or from supplements.

Few amino acids are found naturally in the "free" state. Rather, they must be derived via digestion from complex protein molecules. The technology exists to predigest proteins in order to make amino acids. In addition, chemists are now able to synthesize certain amino acids and/or derive them from bacterial fermentation.

The essential amino acids include the following compounds:

- isoluecine
- leucine
- lysine
- methionine
- phenylalanine
- threonine
- tryptophan
- valine

Phenlyalanine and tryptophan are probably the most important anti-migraine amino acids. Tryptophan can no longer be included as a therapeutic agent. It was pulled off the market as a result of a serious illness that has been associated with its use. Apparently, a Japanese company is responsible for sending a contaminated batch of tryptophan to the United States. This contaminant is the likely culprit behind a disorder known as *Eosinophillic Myalgic Syndrome* (EMS). Tryptophan itself is relatively non-toxic. People are now afraid of using tryptophan, and, to a degree, this is understandable. However, this is also unfortunate. Tryptophan has cured many cases of insomnia, PMS, and, yes, some cases of chronic pain and/or migraine. Whether tryptophan will ever be cleared by the FDA to be placed back on the market remains to be seen. The tryptophan scare need not destroy confidence in the other amino acids especially anti-pain ones such as leucine, tyrosine and phenylalanine.

Phenylalanine is a case in point. As a supplement it can prove invaluable for controlling chronic pain. The DL form, known popularly as *DLPA*, is the most common type available. DLPA is best defined as a natural pain modifier. It acts in concert with the nervous system to control pain. Here is how this works. The brain naturally contains anti-pain compounds similar to opium, except these compounds are up to 100 times more powerful. This means that the human brain has its own special kind of pain killing mechanism which, if properly operating, could obliterate severe pain. The compounds, as discussed previously, are called endorphins and enkephalins. Researchers have discovered that, while endorphins and enkephalins are extremely powerful, their pain killing effects are limited by the fact that they are quickly destroyed. The culprit appears to be an enzyme which inactivates endorphin and enkephalin molecules. This is where DLPA comes in. It actually blocks the ability of the enzyme to deactivate these molecules. This results in a measurable rise in the endorphin/enkephalin levels within the central nervous system.

Chronic pain is commonly associated with endorphin/enkephalin deficiency. In migraine patients, the levels of these substances may be depressed for years. DLPA is by no means a replacement for pain medicines. Its positive effects are gradual, and it may take up to three weeks before benefits are noticed. Yet, it is usually worth the wait. Studies have determined that over 75% of subjects improved in a wide variety of symptoms ranging from pain to depression. The ideal dosage appears to be 1 to 2 grams taken in divided doses.* If you are concerned about overdosing, keep this in mind: DLPA is far less toxic than many of the pills commonly consumed *without concern* including antacids, aspirin, antihistamines, Motrin, Tylenol and laxatives.

Tyrosine Prevents Hormone and Neurotransmitter Deficiency

Tyrosine is an important amino acid although not so much for its anti-pain effects. Its value is a result of the critical role it plays in human physiology. Tyrosine is the precursor for the synthesis of hormones without which human life would be impossible: thyroxin and adrenalin. Without tyrosine, neither can be produced.

Most people are aware that thyroxin (thyroid hormone) is made by the thyroid gland and that adrenalin is produced in the adrenal glands. The thyroid gland is located in the front of the neck just beneath the Adam's apple. The adrenal glands are located on top of the kidneys. It is almost automatic that anyone who has a problem with thyroid and/or adrenal function also has a tyrosine deficiency. Less well known is the fact that the brain produces adrenalin and also a compound known as noradrenalin (norepinephrine), both of which are derived from tyrosine. A deficiency of either of these neurotransmitters increases the vulnerability of the nervous system to painful stimuli. Neurotransmitter deficiency

---

* Warning: Individuals with the hereditary condition *phenylketonuria* must avoid all nutritional supplements containing phenylalanine.

has been associated with chronic pain syndromes, depression, anxiety, insomnia and fatigue.

It is a good idea to boost neurotransmitter levels. An easy way to do this is to take supplemental amino acids, such as tyrosine or phenylalanine, and to increase the consumption of foods rich in these amino acids. These foods include:

- beef
- lamb
- organ meats
- poultry
- cheese
- milk
- wild game

- fish
- eggs
- yogurt
- bee pollen
- sesame seeds

One of the best nutritional cures for depression is tyrosine. This is because tyrosine helps increase brain levels of several neurotransmitters. Two have been mentioned; another is dopamine, a major mood-controlling chemical. Increased dopamine levels can positively affect everything from energy levels to hormone secretion. Dopamine deficiency does occur. This is what happens in Parkinson's disease, and the lack of dopamine is partly responsible for the severe rigidity these patients suffer.

Tyrosine also helps replenish adrenalin levels within the adrenal glands after stress, because stress rapidly depletes adrenalin. One study showed that tyrosine enhances the body's ability to ward off allergic reactions. Can you think of anyone who is depressed, irritable, fatigued and allergic? Tyrosine may well be the answer.

Enzymes

Enzymes are complex protein molecules which serve as the body's work horses. Nearly every chemical process within living organisms depends upon enzymes. The life and function of plants is also entirely dependent upon the enzymes they contain.

A deficiency of enzymes or impaired enzyme function is a contributing factor to many illnesses. The extent of the negative effects depends upon how the enzyme fits into human biochemistry. If a deficiency of digestive enzymes occurs, food is improperly digested which increases the risk for allergic reactions. Incompletely digested food also contributes to the cause of many diseases, including arthritis, colitis, hypoglycemia, lupus, schizophrenia, psoriasis, eczema, diabetes and migraines. It may be necessary for individuals afflicted with these diseases to use digestive enzyme supplements. Often, this will cause a dramatic improvement in the symptoms. Digestion is a key to so many illnesses that it would be accurate to say that any condition will improve if digestion is enhanced.

What we eat, how we eat, how much we eat and how often we eat or drink are the major players in causing ill health or in promoting good health. In many, digestive enzymes may be the missing link between digestive impairment and the promotion of excellent overall health.

Enzymes exist in the human body for more reasons than just digestion. They also act as a sort of garbage disposal system. In other words, they help clean up the cellular wastes. Debris, such as dead cells, tumors and undigested foods, are made up primarily of protein. The only substances that can break down protein are enzymes. Enzymes act in a sense like miniature "pac men," gobbling up the dead protein—that's right, dead protein. Under normal circumstances only dead and diseased tissue is attacked, while healthy tissue is immune to the enzymes' powers.

Enzymes assist the immune system in destroying foreign invaders. Bacteria, viruses, parasites and yeasts are made up primarily of protein. White blood cells contain a considerable amount of enzymes. They use them to digest the microbes once they are engulfed.

It has been discovered that enzymes which are ingested in food can be absorbed into the bloodstream. For years it was believed that this was impossible. The previous thinking was that enzyme molecules were too large to be absorbed or that they, being made of protein, were completely destroyed by stomach acid. However, numerous scientific studies have proven that enzymes can be absorbed intact and that they are still biologically active. Could it be that the actual cells of our bodies will incorporate and utilize these dietary and supplemental enzymes? That is the direction science is pointing.

Enzymes, Allergy and Migraine

Enzymes can be useful in the treatment of migraines by improving digestion, thereby decreasing allergic tendencies. This has been known since the 1930's when Dr. Oelgoetz, an M.D., found that pancreatic enzyme supplements significantly reduced food allergy-related symptoms in his patients. He published his findings in several medical journals. One of the allergy symptoms was migraine. In all cases migraines improved as a result of the enzyme therapy.

When using supplemental enzymes, some caution should be exerted. Pork allergy and, to a lesser degree, beef allergy are fairly common. Therefore, one might wish to utilize a less allergenic source such as lamb pancreas or vegetable-source enzymes. Vegetable enzymes include those made from certain fungi, papain from papayas and also bromelain which is derived from pineapples. Companies which produce quality enzyme products include Klaire Labs, Vitaline, Enzymatic Therapies, Ecological Formulas and Ness.

Not every migraine patient needs to take digestive enzymes. Those who have maldigestion plus migraines definitely need them. The dosage may vary greatly, but a maintenance dose would be two or three capsules after meals.

Fish Oils: Supplement #1 for Migraines

On the surface it seems inconceivable that fats or oils could help cure migraines. One might assume that fats would aggravate the condition by impairing circulation. However, some fats actually improve circulation. The most dominating of these are the fish oils. These are known chemically as *EPA* and *DHA*.

In the old days mothers were known to say, "Fish is brain food." No one could possibly have guessed how prophetic this statement would become. The brain does indeed absorb fish oils. Normally, EPA and DHA are found in brain and nerve tissue.

Fish oils are potent anti-inflammatory agents. Thus, they function to prevent inflammation from occurring in nerve and brain tissue. The retina absorbs fish oils and the oils play a significant role in normal vision. Of all organs in the human body, it appears that the brain has the greatest need for fish oils. Mother was right about it being good for the brain.

The exact function of fish oils in the human brain is unknown. They do act as membrane stabilizers. This is important, since unstable nerve tissue increases the vulnerability for the development of illness, pain or inflammation.

These findings have astounding implications with regard to disorders of the nervous system. The inference is that brain tissue rich in fish oils is more stable against noxious stimuli which might damage or irritate the central nervous system. Could this also mean that the same stimulus which would have provoked a migraine no longer will if the brain contains a higher percentage of fatty acids from fish oils? Only further research will tell.

Fish oils exert several other positive effects upon the circulatory system. They help improve blood flow, and this effect can be dramatic. They assist in the healing of damaged arterial walls and prevent healthy ones from degenerating. Hardening of the arteries, a plague of modern civilization, is non-existent in Eskimos who eat fatty fish. Fish oils prevent blood clots, thereby diminishing the incidence of stroke, and they all but eliminate sludging of the blood. Such sludging is seen in migraines as well as in lung disease, heart disease, claudication, high blood pressure, Raynaud's disease, diabetes and peripheral vascular disease.

Fish oils are Nature's blood thinners par excellence. They do this job better than aspirin and without the side effects.* This blood-thinning ef-

---

*Individuals taking aspirin, Coumadin, heparin or other blood thinners who wish to take fish oil supplements must do so only while under a doctor's care.

fect is easy to explain. It appears that the platelets, the cells responsible for blood clotting, have a preference for EPA and DHA similar to that seen in brain cells. Platelets rapidly incorporate fish oils into their membranes. The oils somehow alter platelet function to keep them from becoming excessively sticky. Having sticky platelets can be a dangerous thing, especially if there is a family history or a current history of circulatory disease, blood clots or stroke.

All of these effects combined make fish oils one of the top antimigraine nutrients. Science is proving this. Researchers have found that fish oils reduce the inflammation of migraines during the migraine crisis. In the right dose, these oils lessen the severity of migraine attacks by 50%. Just think what can be accomplished preventively by religiously consuming fish oils every day. The result will undoubtedly be better health, and a reduction in the severity and frequency of migraines is likely.

Fish oils can be added to the diet simply by eating fish rich in these oils. Fish containing the highest amount of EPA/DHA are those found in cold water, and they exist both in fresh and salt water. This makes sense. Fish living in frigid waters need insulation, and fat serves this function nicely. Those living in the coldest water, such as the arctic, have the most fatty insulation and, therefore, contain the highest amounts of fish oils. Top sources include:

mackerel
salmon (especially Atlantic)
trout (especially lake)
sardines
herring
abalone
anchovies
tuna (especially albacore)
whitefish
haddock
cod

Other fish which contain considerable amounts of fish oils include:

sablefish
sturgeon
shrimp
crab
bluefish

Migraine patients should eat more of these fish, that is if they are not allergic to them. It would be a good idea to eat fish rich in EPA/DHA at least twice per week as a means of preventing migraine attacks. The existence of sticky platelets increases the risk for migraine attacks. Unstick them the natural way with fish oils, not with aspirin or other potentially damaging drugs.

Another way to get fish oils is via supplements. EPA/DHA supplements have become popular, particularly in the last decade. They were first introduced by a British company under the trade name *MaxEPA*. Of late, fish oil products have fallen out of vogue as a result of bad publicity. It appears that certain companies, in an effort to get on the bandwagon, have produced and marketed inferior products which have rated poorly when tested and scrutinized by the scientific community. The real scare came when scientists found that some of these products actually caused an increase in cholesterol levels. Further research determined that fish oils, like many oils, have a tendency to become rancid. It is likely that this rancidity caused mild toxicity, and this was manifested by an unexpected rise in cholesterol levels. There is another problem with low-grade fish oil products. Many are made from very large fish; some of these creatures have lived in the oceans for decades. Such fish are more likely to contain high levels of toxic chemicals which can leach into the supplements, since many of these chemicals are fat soluble.

For these reasons the fish oil supplement recommended in this book is Kyolic-EPA. This product is made from sardines, one of the richest sources of EPA. Sardines are far less likely to contain fat-soluble toxic chemicals than are larger fish.

In addition, rancidity is not a concern with Kyolic-EPA. This product contains one of Nature's most potent antioxidants—Kyolic garlic. The garlic keeps the fish oils from turning rancid, a common problem which occurs when these oils are exposed to the elements, i.e. air, light and heat. Plus, like fish oils, Kyolic garlic inhibits platelet aggregation.

It has been known for years that certain oils, notably the polyunsaturates, easily become rancid, especially if they are heated. The only thing that stops the rancidity is to add preservatives. This is why commercial manufacturers, after producing refined vegetable oils, commonly add the synthetic antioxidants *BHT* and *BHA*. These potent antioxidants prevent the oils from turning rancid during storage, helping prolong shelf life. Unfortunately, these preservatives may themselves be toxic and would be inappropriate for adding to a "healthfood" supplement. Rather, we must turn to natural antioxidants and preservatives such as garlic and vitamin E. Both are found in Kyolic-EPA.

All this is important, because rancid oils are unfit for human consumption. Such oils cause digestive upset, aggravate existing illnesses or may even cause disease. How can you tell if a fish oil product is rancid? Simple—by the smell. The more fishy the odor is, the more rancid it will be. Prolonged after-taste may also be an indication of rancidity. However, don't let this scare you from using fish oils. People freely use aspirin as a blood thinner. Undoubtedly, fish oils are far safer.

GLA: The Other Anti-Migraine Fatty Acid

GLA (gamma linolenic acid) is an essential fatty acid. In contrast, fish oils have not, as of yet, been classified as essential. An essential fatty acid is one which is, as the name implies, essential to life itself. This means that without GLA human life could not exist. Disease and death can result from a prolonged deficiency. This is largely because GLA and other essential fatty acids must be obtained from the diet and cannot be made within the human body.

Most Americans are deficient in this crucial nutrient. One reason is that we are simply not getting enough of it in the diet. Another is that many commonly consumed substances destroy or block the utilization of GLA. A list of substances and conditions which negatively affect GLA includes:

birth control pills
alcohol
cigarette smoke
chewing tobacco
chlorinated water
deep fried foods
junk foods
partially hydrogenated or hydrogenated oils
radiation
toxic chemicals
yeast infections
diabetes
arthritis
cancer
chronic viral illness

In addition, zinc and B-6 deficiency make it all but impossible for the body to utilize GLA; over 60% of Americans are deficient in both zinc and B-6. Symptoms of GLA deficiency include dry skin, eczema, brittle or dry hair, hair loss, easy bruising, delayed growth, brittle nails, excessive thirst, increased susceptibility to infection, infertility, dry mouth and/or eyes, thick saliva, delayed wound healing, PMS and fibrocystic breasts.

What does all this have to do with headaches? Remember, the brain is made up primarily of fats which occur biochemically in the form of fatty acids. Among the most important fatty acids in brain function are the ones in which Americans are most commonly deficient—GLA, fish oils and lecithin. GLA is easily absorbed into the brain. It helps stabilize the nerves, making them less susceptible to disease and inflammation. It has another powerful effect unrelated to the brain. It helps diminish PMS, thus reducing the occurrence of PMS-induced headaches. GLA should form a part of the anti-migraine nutritional regimen, especially in the case of menstruating women. A dose of 9 to 12 capsules per day should be sufficient (see Appendix C).

That drugs are usually far more potent in killing headache pain than nutrients cannot be denied. The nutrients described in this chapter are not meant to be equivalents for replacing pain-controlling drugs. Nutrients are useful primarily for the prevention of pain, not for its treatment. Always keep this in mind when using nutrients in the treatment of migraines.

CHAPTER 8
Conclusion

Migraine headaches can be cured. So can other kinds of headaches. It is possible to live without headache pain. In a majority of instances migraines can be eliminated by determining the cause and treating it.

Migraines due to food allergies are the easiest to cure. All that needs to be done is to determine what the allergies are and avoid them. Foods have more to do with causing headaches than chemicals, toxins, infections or disease. There is no one universal list of migraine-provoking foods. Each person's food list will vary. However, cheeses, wine, pork, cocoa, corn, shrimp, wheat, eggs and coffee are commonly implicated. In addition, every person with allergic migraines has a different pattern in regard to the type of headache he/she has. Some get headaches immediately after eating the offending food, while in others, the headaches occur days after the incident. The pain may last anywhere from a few hours to as long as a week. As hard as it is to believe, there are actually people who have daily headaches. These can persist for weeks or even months and are often entirely a result of consuming allergic foods. Substances other than foods which provoke headaches include food additives, alcoholic beverages, industrial chemicals and fumes.

It is debilitating, as most anyone can imagine, to experience frequent or constant headaches. Not only do the headaches cause pain, but they actually fatigue the sufferer both physically and emotionally. They place a strain upon those who care, who hate to see a loved one writhe in constant

114

pain. Yet, no one suffers like the one who lives with the pain day in and day out.

This book was written to be used as a tool to solve the migraine dilemma. The goal is to eliminate headaches, reduce suffering and improve lifestyle. At a minimum, it was written to help reduce the frequency of this terrible illness. People with migraines know that any improvement is worthwhile. Why not attempt to achieve as much improvement as is possible?

A great deal can be accomplished by curing headaches. As a result, a person's entire life is changed. A life of pain becomes one of pleasure. Sick leave is decreased, productivity is enhanced and vitality is improved. Overall health is greatly accelerated, and the individual becomes more energetic, not to speak of having an improved mental outlook and a happier personality. Life moves from drudgery to a dream come true. Getting rid of this paralyzing illness lifts a phenomenal burden, and the journey through life will become far more pleasurable.

This book makes it clear that there is no need for migraine patients to resign themselves to "living with the pain." Some so called experts in the field would have it believed that migraines are largely incurable. On the contrary, many measures can be taken. This book lists proven remedies. It provides other options which have been found to be valuable in a clinical setting.

However, it is realized that the methods and treatments outlined in this book are not for everyone. Some will fail to try this approach because of skepticism. Questions raised by skeptics might include, "Why don't other doctors use these methods if they are so effective?" or, "Why would doctors say there are no cures if there really are some?" Many skeptics will question the concept of food allergies as the primary cause of migraines. Others might find it hard to believe that nutrients could be used to replace drugs. These questions and concerns can easily be rebutted. All one has to do is review the bibliography. Numerous scientific articles supporting the claims in this book are listed. The migraine patient should, at a minimum, know one thing: *Migraines do have a cause, and a cure is likely to result if that cause is found and effectively treated.* If nothing else, remember this: investigate anything with potential. People take this attitude in other areas of life, including business, sports and pleasure. Why not with health?

It is true that many illnesses other than allergies cause or worsen headaches. The list includes infection, PMS, chemical sensitivity, muscle tension, high blood pressure, hypothyroidism, adrenal gland disorders and the more serious conditions such as brain tumors. Life-threatening causes of migraines account for a relatively small percentage of cases.

Rather than working toward determining the cause, most people resort to the use of chemicals and drugs which act only to treat the symptoms of headaches. Drugs are a cover-up. While they may give immediate relief, they do nothing to treat the cause. The list of drugs commonly used for headaches includes aspirin, Bufferin, Excedrin, Motrin, Tylenol, Cafergot, Midrin, Empirin, Valium, Xanax and Inderal. Some people take drugs—aspirin for example—like they are eating candy and think nothing of it. They should give it thought, since the risks of toxicity to human tissues run high at these elevated drug dosages. Plus, drugs may increase the susceptibility to migraines via the physiological damage they perpetrate.

On the positive side, drugs do kill pain. If they are eliminated, what remains for controlling the pain? There are few magic pills in nutrition. That's one reason drugs are so popular, because people often feel the effects immediately.

Yet, the quick fix approach does nothing to achieve a long-term cure. Rather, it is somewhat like patching up a junky automobile to keep it running a few more miles. This is a haphazard approach. When it comes to the human body, the quick-fix approach can ultimately prove damaging. By neglecting the cause, the illness is often prolonged. Thus, the potential for physiological damage is increased. The sooner the problem is diagnosed and corrected, the better off the patient will be. Drug dependency, whether to narcotics or over the counter pain killers, is a negative situation, the negative effects being both physical and mental. Getting off the drugs is an important step in the migraine cure process.

Good nutrition and prevention through food allergy removal can produce unbelievable results. Isn't it remarkable that a person could be cured of migraines just by avoiding certain foods? Because of this approach, people who have had migraines for decades and who have searched all over this nation are now living free of pain.

Twenty million people have migraines. As many as 45 million Americans have experienced a headache of some sort. That's nearly one fourth of the population. People of fame, past and present, have suffered the illness. They include St. Gregory, Chopin, Charles Darwin, Sigmund Freud, Thomas Jefferson and George Bernard Shaw. Mr. Shaw, the noted British historian, a witty character, confronted another migraine sufferer, the renowned Norwegian North Pole explorer, Fridjof Nansen. He said, "Mr. Nansen, have you found a cure for headaches?" Mr. Nansen replied, "No," then Mr. Shaw said, "Astonishing . . . you have spent your life trying to discover the North Pole, which nobody cares about, and you have never attempted to discover a cure for headaches which every living person is crying aloud for?" Mr. Shaw and many other famous individuals probably searched in every way they could for relief or cure. Ironically, the cure was more obvious and simple than any of these brilliant men could comprehend.

One need not search the far reaches of the globe for a migraine cure. There is no need to make a valiant effort to glean through the years of accumulated medical research in order to search for some missing link. The cure is within reach: it is what we put in our mouths that causes the vast majority of migraines. Whether that be a cigarette, medicine, alcoholic beverage, coffee or food, this is where it all begins.

It has been said that the origin of illness is largely a consequence of how much we abuse our bodies. The most common abuses involve dietary habits or, more descriptively, habits which control what goes into our bodies. Eating to an excess is one form of abuse. Consuming substances known to be toxic, like cigarette smoke, is another. There is a third abuse, one which is entirely unintentional and one which is difficult to explain. It is the consumption of allergic foods which under any other circumstances would be good for the body. Is eating broccoli or carrots bad for you? It can be, but *only if you are allergic to them.*

Headaches are second only to colds as the common complaint in doctors' offices. In the U.S.A. alone over four billion dollars are spent each year in attempt to alleviate headache pain. A great deal of this is spent in futility, since most therapies do little more than camouflage the pain. Why wouldn't a person accept a trial of medicine when he/she is told, "It's only nerves" or "You're under too much stress." Fortunately, however, money and time can be spent more judiciously, with better results, permanent cure and less strain over the long haul.

John Mansfield, M.D., a pioneer of allergy research in Britain, states in the conclusion of his book, *Migraine and the Allergy Connection,* "*Food allergy plays the greatest single part in the causation of this* (migraine) *disease.*" Mansfield is one of many modern researchers convinced that migraines are due to food allergies and that proper diagnosis and treatment will lead to a cure.

The alternative treatments for migraine need not be bizarre or unscientific. They should be based on a sound, scientific and clinical model. The prescribed treatment methods are scientific and are also effective. It is hoped that this book offers solutions for this pervasive problem once and for all.

APPENDIX A

Foods Containing WHEAT:

beer
biscuits
bouillon cubes
bread: corn, gluten, graham, pumpernickel, white, rye, oat, soy
cake
candy
candy bars
cereals
chocolate
cookies
crackers
doughnuts
flour
gin
gravies
ice cream cones
macaroni
matzos
mayonnaise
muffins
noodles
Ovaltine

pancakes, waffles
pizza
pies
popovers
Postum
pretzels
puddings
rolls
sausage, cold meats
synthetic pepper
whiskies
yeast

Foods Containing EGGS:

baking powders
Bavarian cream
bouillon
breads, breaded foods
cakes
candies
consommes
cookies
creamed pies
coquettes
custards
doughnuts
French toast
fritters
frostings
Hollandaise sauce
ice cream
icings
macaroni
macaroons
malted cocoa drinks
marshmallows
mayonnaise
meat loaf
meringues
noodles
omelets
pancakes
pasta
pretzels

puddings
salad dressing
sausage
sherbet
souffles
soups
tartar sauce
timbales
waffles
wine

Foods Containing SOY BEAN:

bread
cake
candies
cereal
cheese (processed)
cold cuts
flour
fried foods (home and commercial)
gravies
hamburger helper
hamburger patties
ice cream
iced milk
margarine
mayonnaise
milk substitutes
non-dairy products
nuts
packaged mixes
pastas
pastries
potato chips
rolls
salad dressing
sausage
sherbet
shortenings (liquid and solid)
soy sauce
vegetable oil
wieners
Worchestershire Sauce

Foods containing MILK:

au gratin foods
baking powder biscuits
Bavarian cream
bisques
bologna
bread
breakfast or diet drinks
butter
buttermilk
butter sauces
cakes
candy
chocolate drinks
chowders
cookies
cream
cheese
doughnuts
eggs (scrambled)
flour mixtures: biscuit, muffin, cake, pancake, waffle, pudding
gravies
hot cakes
ice cream
mashed potatoes
malted milk
meat loaf
omelet
popovers
protein powders
salad dressings
sherbets
soda crackers
souffles
soup

Foods Containing PORK:

bacon
bacon drippings
bakery products
candy bars
canned meat
Chinese food
chitterlings (chitlins)

gelatin, jello etc.
ham
ice cream (mono/diglycerides)
lard
liverwurst
lunch meat
margarine
mashed potatoes (instant)
mayonnaise
Mexican food (tortillas etc.)
mincemeat
non dairy cream, Coffee Mate, etc.
pancake mixes
pickled pigs feet
Polynesian food
pork and beans
pork rinds
potato chips, Fritos etc.
pre-breaded frozen foods (frozen seafood and fish)
puddings
salad dressings
salads
sausage
shortening
Spam
vegetable stock
Vienna sausage
wieners

Foods Containing YEAST:

bacon
barbecue sauce
bread
buns
butter
cake and cake mix
canned fruit and vegetables
cheese (all kinds)
chili peppers
condiments
cookies
crackers
flour enriched with vitamins from yeast
French dressing

frozen or canned citrus fruit juices
Gerber's oatmeal
ham
horseradish
jam
jelly
ketchup
malted products (cereal, candy, malted milk drinks)
mayonnaise
meat fried in cracker crumbs
milk fortified with vitamins from yeast
mince pie
molasses
mushrooms
olives
pastries
pickles
preserves
pretzels
rolls, home made and canned
root beer
salad dressing
sauerkraut
sour cream
syrup
tomato sauce
truffels
vitamin tablets/capsules
vinegar (apple, pear, grape and distilled)
alcohol (whiskey, wine, brandy, rum, vodka, beer and gin)

Foods Containing COTTONSEED OIL:

breaded frozen foods
breads, rolls and buns
cake, cookie and pastry mixes
candies
deep fried foods
doughnuts
foods processed by commercial frying and baking
frozen pizza
lard or solid shortening
margarine
mayonnaise
microwave popcorn

pastries, pies and cakes
salad oils
sardines (may be packed in cottonseed oil)
snack foods of all types (chips, crackers, cookies)

Sources of Added NITRATES in Food:

bacon
bologna
bratwurst
chipped beef
corn dogs
corned beef
ham
head cheese
hot dogs
jerky
liverwurst
pastrami
pickled pigs feet
pork and beans
salami
sausage
sliced chicken and turkey breast (some)
smoked salmon (and other smoked fish)
smoked turkey
Spam
turkey bologna
turkey ham
turkey salami

Note: Even if one is not allergic to nitrates or the foods containing them, it is possible to get a headache due to the nitrate-induced chemical toxicity of the blood.

Foods containing SULFITES:

baked goods
batters
breadings
canned fruits
canned vegetables
coffee
cole slaw
cornstarch
dried fruits

fish products, including fresh fish
frozen vegetables
fruit drinks
fruit salad
fruit toppings
gelatins
gravies and sauces
guacamole
hard candy
instant tea
jams and jellies
jarred fruits
olives
pancake syrup
pickles
pie fillings
potato chips
potato salad
puddings
relishes
salad dressings
soups (canned or dried)
tortilla chips
vinegars
white and brown sugar

Foods Containing MSG:

Accent or Lawry's seasoning
bacon bits
baking mixes
batters
beef jerky
bouillon cubes
bread stuffings
breaded deep fried foods
breaded/frozen foods
breadings
brown or creamy gravies and sauces
canned meats
canned tuna (Chicken of the Sea, Bumble Bee and Geisha brands)
cheese dips and sauces
cheese puffs
Chef Boyardee products
chicken and beef spreads (Swanson and Underwood brands)

chili, canned (Hormel)
Chinese food, canned
chip dip
clam chowder
corn or tortilla chips
croutons
dry roasted nuts (Planters)
frozen dinners (Swansons, Morton, Weight Watchers, Lean Cuisine)
frozen pizza
frozen pot pies
frozen potato products (French fries, Tater Tots)
gelatins
packed noodles or pasta
potato chips
processed and cured meats, (hot dogs, bologna, bacon, etc.)
processed cheeses
processed poultry products
puddings
relishes
salad dressings
salt substitutes
seasonings
soft candies
soups, canned or dried
soy sauce
stew, canned

Foods Containing SALICYLATES:

almonds
apples
apricots
blackberries
cherries
cloves
cucumbers and pickles
currants
gooseberries
grapes and raisins
mint flavors
nectarines
oranges
peaches
peppermint
prunes, plums

raspberries
spearmint
strawberries
tea, all varieties
tomatoes
wines
wine vinegars
wintergreen

APPENDIX B

List of Foods
Evaluated for Allergies
Via Food Intolerance Test

Seafood

clam
crab
lobster
oyster
scallop
shrimp

Fish

bass
carp
catfish
caviar
cod
flounder
haddock
halibut
herring
lake perch
lake trout
mackerel
orange roughy
pike
red snapper
salmon
sardine
sea perch
shark
smelt
sole
swordfish
tuna

Poultry

chicken
chicken egg yolk
chicken egg white

duck
pheasant
turkey

Red Meat

beef
lamb
pork

Milk Products

bleu cheese
butter
buttermilk
cheddar cheese
cottage cheese
cow's milk
goat's milk
mozzarella cheese
Parmesan cheese
provolone cheese
Swiss cheese
yogurt

Grains

barley
millet
oats
rice
rye
wheat
wheat bran

Fruit

apple
apricot
avocado
banana
blackberry
blueberry
cantaloupe
cherry
coconut
cranberry

date
fig
grape
grapefruit
honey dew melon
lemon
lime
mango
nectarine
olive
orange
papaya
peach
pear
pineapple
plum (prune)
pomegranate
raspberry
rhubarb
strawberry
tomato
watermelon

Vegetables

alfalfa sprouts
artichoke
asparagus
beet
broccoli
Brussels sprouts
cabbage
carrot
cauliflower
celery
chicory
chestnut
corn
cucumber
eggplant
endive
garden (bell) pepper
garlic
green bean
horseradish

kale
lettuce
okra
onions
parsley
parsnip
pimento
pumpkin
radish
rutabaga
spinach
squash
string beans
Swiss chard
turnip
watercress
water chestnuts

Nuts and Seeds

almond
black walnut
Brazil nut
cashew
chestnuts
English walnut
filbert
pecan
pistachio
safflower seed (oil)
sesame seed (oil)
sunflower seed

Spices

allspice
anise seed
basil
bay leaf
black pepper
caraway seed
chili pepper
chives
cinnamon
clove
cumin seed

curry
dill seed
ginger
marjoram
nutmeg
oregano
paprika
peppermint (spearmint)
rosemary
sage
thyme
turmeric

Sweeteners

beet sugar
cane sugar
honey
malt
maple sugar
molasses
Nutra Sweet
saccharin
sorbitol
sorghum

Beans and Legumes

bean sprouts
black eyed peas
carob
chick pea
kidney beans
lentil
lima bean
mung bean
peanut
pinto bean
soybean
split pea

Miscellaneous

baker's yeast
brewer's yeast
buckwheat

cocoa
coffee
cola
cotton seed oil
food dyes
frog legs
gelatin
hops
MSG
mushroom
potato
salicylate
sulfites
sweet potato
tapioca
tea
tobacco
vanilla
yam

APPENDIX C

Additive-Free Foods

Product	Company
Dried Fruits, Jams, Wild Nuts, Sauces	American Spoon Foods 1668 Clarion Avenue Petoskey, Michigan 49770 (800) 222-5886
Coleman's Organic Beef	Coleman's Nitrate-Free Hot Dogs and Other Meats P.O. Box 170457A Denver, Colorado 80217 (Available in fine health food stores)
All-Natural Hazelnuts, Honey-Roasted Hazelnuts and Hazel-Nut Butter	Henry's Farms 1216 E. Henry Road Newberry, Oregon 97132 (503) 538-5244
Honey and Fruit Toppings and Honey Nut Butters	Oregon Apiaries Newberg, Oregon 97132 (503) 538-8546
Organic Buffalo (bison) Meat	U.S. Bison Company W 11282 Wildlife Road Withee, Wisconsin 54498 (800) 225-7457
Additive-Free Frozen Dinners (Taste great too!)	Oven Poppers 405 Spruce Street Manchester, New Hampshire 03103 Call collect (603) 644-3773

Nutritional Products

These supplements are of the highest quality and are free of additives and preservatives:

Primrose Oil (GLA)	Biotech Box 1992 Fayetteville, Arizona 72702 (800) 356-4791

Fish Oils, (EPA/DHA), Kyodophilus, odor-free Kyolic Garlic	"Kyolic-EPA" Wakunaga Corporation Mission Viejo, California (800) 421-2998 (Available at fine health food stores)
Ginger Root	Nature's Way Springville, Utah 84663 (Available at fine health food stores)
Feverfew (freeze-dried, standardized extract)	Cardiovascular Research Concord, California Mail Order: (800) 243-5242
Bilberry Extract (for eye strain)	Enzymatic Therapies Green Bay, Wisconsin (Available at fine health food stores)
Chromium Picolinate, P-5-P (Pyridoxal-5-Phosphate)	Klaire Labs Carlsbad, California Mail Order: (800) 243-5242 (Available at fine health food stores)
Magnesium Taurate	Ecological Formulas Concord, California Mail Order: (800) 243-5242
Digestive Enzymes (hypoallergenic, Lamb-source)	Ecological Formulas Klaire Labs Mail Order: (800) 243-5242
Soy and Wheat Germ Oil-Free Vitamin E	AC Grace Co. Big Sandy, Texas Mail Order: (800) 243-5242

OsteoGuard (for strong bones and joints)

Advanced Medical Nutrition
Hayward, California
(800) 243-5242

APPENDIX D

Physicians and Laboratories

The following is a list of physicians skilled at performing allergy testing as described in this book for diagnosing allergy-induced migraine:

Cass Igram, D.O.
6399 Wilshire Blvd Suite 701
Los Angeles, California 90048
(213) 655-5602

Optimum Health Center
850 Marsh Street, Suite C
Valparaiso, Indiana 46383
(219) 462-3377

Menner Chiropractic
1655 Rand
Lake Zurich, Illinois 60047
(708) 540-6060

Norman Miller, D.O.
516 S. Main Street
Middlebury, Indiana 46540
(219) 825-9124

Beverly Joseph, D.O.
1056 Fourth Street
Des Moines, Iowa 50314
(515) 288-3507

Richard Hrdlicka, MD
302 Randall
Geneva, Illinois 60134
(708) 232-1900

Laboratories and Pharmacy

Food Allergy and
Cellular Vitamin Testing

Nutritional Testing Laboratories
Continental Towers II
1701 Golf Road, Suite 606
Rolling Meadows, Illinois 60008
(708) 640-1377

Leaky Gut Syndrome,
Secretory IgA

Diagnos-Techs
P.O. Box 58948
Seattle, Washington 98138
(800) 878-3787

Hair Analysis,
Toxic Metal Screen

Doctor's Data
P.O. Box 111
West Chicago, Illinois 60185
(800) 323-2784

Standardized Thyroid

College Pharmacy
833 N. Tejon Street
Colorado Springs, Colorado 80903
(800) 748-2263

BIBLIOGRAPHY

Abraham, G.E., and M.M. Lubran. 1981. Serum and red cell magnesium levels in patients with premenstrual tension. *American Journal of Clinical Nutrition* 34:2364-2366.

Anderson, R.A., Bryden, N.A., et al. 1985. Chromium supplementation of human subjects. *Nutrition Research* suppl. 1:560-63.

Ammann, A.J., and R. Long. 1970. Selective IgA deficiency and autoimmunity. *Clin. Exp. Immunol.* 7:833-38.

Ammann, A.J., and R. Long. 1971. Selective IgA deficiency: representation of 30 cases and a review of the literature. *Medicine* 50:223-36.

Arora, R.B., et al. 1971. Anti-inflammatory studies on curcuma longa (turmeric). *Ind. J. Med. Res.* 59(8):1289.

Bali, L. 1978. Vitamin C and migraine: a case report. *N.E.J.M.* (letter to the editor) Aug. 17, p. 364.

Barnes, B.O., and C.W. Barnes. 1972. *Heart Attack Rareness in Thyroid Treated Patients.* Charles C. Thomas, Springfield, Ill.

Barnes, B.O., and L. Galton. 1976. *Hypothyroidism: The Unsuspected Illness.* Thomas Y. Crowell Co., New York.

Bernstein, I.D., et al. 1968. Absorption of antigens from the gastrointestinal tract. *Int. Arch. Allergy Applied Immuno.* 33:521-29.

Bille, B. 1962. Migraine in school children. *Acta paediat.* suppl. 51:136.

Bjarnason, I., Ward, K., et al. 1984. The leaky gut of alcoholism: possible route of entry for toxic compounds. *Lancet* 28, Jan.

Bjarnason, I., et al. 1984. Intestinal permeability and inflammation in rheumatoid arthritis: effects of non-steroidal anti-inflammatory drugs. *Lancet* Nov. 24, p. 42.

Bjarnason, I., et al. 1987. Blood and protein loss via small intestinal inflammation induced by non-steroidal anti-inflammatory drugs. *Lancet* 2:711-715.

Blau, J.N. 1984. Towards a definition of migraine headache. *Lancet* 1:444-45.

Bock, S.A., and C.D. May. 1983. Adverse reactions to food caused by sensitivity. In Middleton, E., Jr., Reed, C.E., and Ellis, E.F., eds.: *Allergy Principles and Practice.* C.V. Mosby Co. St. Louis, Mo. pp. 1415-25.

Bogduk, N. 1980. The anatomy of occipital neuralgia. *Clin. Exp. Neuro.* 17:167.

Bourcher, R.C., Pare, P.D., and J.C. Hogg. 1979. Relationship between airway hyperactivity and hyperpermeability in ascaris sensitive monkeys. *J. Allergy Clin. Immunol.* 64:197-201.

Breneman, J.C. 1978. *Basics of Food Allergy.* Charles C. Thomas, Springfield, Ill.

Bryan, W.T.K., and M.P. Bryan. 1971. Cytotoxic reaction in the diagnosis of food allergy. *Otolaryngol. Clin. N. Am.* 4:523-34.

Buckley, R.H., et al. 1969. Correlation of milk precipitins with IgA deficiency. *N.E.J.M.* 281:465-69.

Buist, R. 1984. *Food Intolerance: What It Is and How to Cope With It.* Harper & Rowe, Sydney, Australia.

Busse, W.W., Koop, D.E., and E. Middleton. 1984. Flavonoid modulation of human neutrophil function. *J. Allergy Clin. Immunol.* 73:801-9.

Caradoc-Davies, T.H. 1984. Nonsteroidal anti-inflammatory drugs, arthritis, and gastrointestinal bleeding in elderly in-patients. *Age and Aging* 13:295-98.

Clark, D. 1948. The endocrine approach to the treatment of allergy. *Ann. Western Med. Surg.* 22(9):404-407.

Clausen, J. 1988. Chromium induced clinical improvement in symptomatic hypoglycemia. *Bio. T. Elem. Res.* 17:229-36.

Congon, P.J., and W.I. Forsythe. 1979. Migraine and childhood; a study of 300 children. *Develop. Med. Child. Neurol.* 21:209-16.

Couch, J.R., and R.S. Hassenein. 1977. Platelet aggregability in migraine. *Neurology* 27:643.

Cousins, N. 1979. *Anatomy of an Illness.* W.W. Norton & Co., New York.

Crabbe', P.A., Carbonaro, A.O., and J.F. Heremans. 1965. The normal human intestinal mucosa as a major source of plasma cells containing IgA. *Int. Acad. Path.* 14(3):235-39.

Crabbe', P.A., Bazin, H., Eyssen, H., et al. 1968. The normal flora as a major stimulus for proliferation of plasma cells synthesizing IgA in the gut. *Int. Arch. Allergy* 34:362-75.

Crayton, J.W., Stone, T., and G.G. Stein. 1981. Epilepsy precipitated by food sensitivity: report of a case with double-blind placebo controlled assessment. *Clin. Electroencephalogr.* 12(4):192-8.

D'Anglejan-Chatillon, J., et al. 1989. Migraine—a risk factor for dissection of cervical arteries. *J.A.M.A.* Vol. 263 No. 17.

Dalton, K. 1975. Food intake prior to a migraine attack: study of 2,313 spontaneous attacks. *Headache* 15(3):188-93.

Degowin, E.L. 1932. Allergic migraine: a review of sixty cases. *J. Allergy* 3:557-66.

Delespesse, G., et al. 1976. Cellular aspect of selective IgA deficiency. *Clin. Exp. Immunol.* 24:273-79.

Deluca, L.M., et al. 1986. Vitamin A and the liver. *Prog. Liver Dis.* 8:81-98.

Diamond, S.D. 1988. *Hope for your Headache Problem.* Revised ed. International Univ. Press, Madison.

Donovan, E.W. 1985. *Essentials of Pathophysiology.* Macmillan Publishing Co., New York.

Drummond, P.D., and J.W. Lance. 1983. Extracranial vascular changes and the source of pain in migraine headache. *Ann. Neuro.* 13:32.

Eaton, C.D. 1954. Co-existence of hypothyroidism with diabetes mellitus. *J. Mich. Med. Soc.* 53:1101.

Egger, J., Carter, C.M., Wilson, J., et al. 1983. Is migraine food allergy? A double-blind controlled trial of oligoantigenic diet treatment. *Lancet* 2:865-868.

Egger, J., Carter, M., Soothill, J.F., et al. 1989. Oligoantigenic diet treatment of children with epilepsy and migraine. *J. Pediatrics* 114(1):51-57.

Ensminger, A.H., et al. 1983. *Foods and Nutrition Encyclopedia*. Vol. 1&2, Pergus Press, Clovis, CA.

Eyermann, C.H. 1931. Allergic headache. *J. Allergy* 2:106-12.

Ferrari, A., and E. Sternieri. 1990. Dietary headaches through the centuries. *Funct. Neurol.* 5:79-84.

Fredericks, C., and H. Goodman. 1969. *Low Blood Sugar and You.* Constellations International, New York.

Freed, D.L.F. 1978. Mucotractive effect of lectin. *Lancet* 1:585-6.

Freed, D.L.F., and R.J. Cooper. 1977. Cytotoxicity of bread and soya protein in tissue culture. *Lancet* 2:371.

Giacovazzo, M., and P. Martelletti. 1989. Letter to the editor. *Ann. Allergy* 63:255.

Glover, V., Snadler, M., Grant, E., et al. 1977. Transitory decrease in platelet monoamine oxidase activity during migraine attacks. *Lancet* 1:391-93.

Gold, M. 1982. Significant number of depressives may have hypothyroidism. *Family Practice News* Nov. 1.

Goltman, M.A. 1936. Mechanism of migraine. *J. Allergy* 7:351.

Gotze, H. 1975. Enteropancreatic circulation of digestive enzymes as a conservation mechanism. *Nature* 257:607-9.

Graham, J.R., and H.G. Wolff. 1937. Mechanisms of migraine headache and action of ergotamine tartrate. *Illinois Med. J.* 99:210.

Grant, E.G. 1965. Relation of arterioles in the endometrium to headache from oral contraceptives. *Lancet* 1:1143-44.

Grant, E.G., Albuquerque, M., Steiner, T.J., et al. 1978. Oral contraceptives, smoking and ergotamine in migraine. *Current Concepts in Migraine Research.* R. Greene, ed. Raven Press, New York.

Grant, E.G. 1979. Food allergies and migraine. *Lancet* 1:966-69.

Gunn, C.C., and W.E. Milbrandt. 1977. Utilizing trigger points. *Osteopathic Physician* Mar.

Hanington, E. 1971. Migraine. *Trans. Med. Soc.* 87:32.

Hanington, E., Jones, R.J., Arness, J.A., et al. 1981. Migraine: a platelet disorder. *Lancet* 2:720-23.

Harrison, D.P. 1986. Copper as a factor in the dietary precipitation of migraine. *Headache* 26(5):248-50.

Havsteen, B. 1983. Flavonoids, a class of natural products of high pharmacological potency. *Biochem. Pharm.* 32:1121-8.

Heaney, R.P., and R.R. Recker. 1986. Distribution of calcium absorption in middle aged women. *Am. J. Clin. Nutr.* 43:229-305.

Heatley, R.V., Denburg, J.A., Bayer, N., et al. 1982. Increased plasma histamine levels in migraine patients. *Clin. Allergy* 12:145-49.

Henderson, W.R., and N.H. Raskin. 1972. Hot-dog headache: individual susceptibility to nitrite. *Lancet* 2:1162.

Hollander, D., and H. Tarnawski. 1985. Aging-associated increase in intestinal absorption of macromolecules. *Gerontology* 31:133-137.

Horrobin, D.F. 1981. The importance of gamma-linolenic acid and prostaglandin E-1 in human nutrition and medicine. *J. Holistic Med.* 3(2):11839.

Hurxthal, L.M. 1934. Blood cholesterol and thyroid disease. *Arch. Int. Med.* 53:825.

Jameson, S., Arfors, K., et al. 1985. Pain relief and selenium balance in patients with connective tissue disease and osteoarthrosis: a double blind selenium tocopherol supplementation study. *Nutrition Research* suppl. 1:391-397.

Jennings, I.W. 1970. *Vitamins in Endocrine Metabolism.* Charles C. Thomas, Springfield, Ill.

Johns, D.R. 1986. Migraine provoked by aspartame. *N.E.J.M.* 315:456.

Kabacoff, B.L., et al. 1963. Absorption of chymotryspin from the intestinal tract. *Nature* 199:815.

Kailin, E.W., and A. Hastings. 1966. Electromyographic evidence of DDT-induced myoasthenia. *Medical Annals District Columbia* 35:237.

Kailin, E.W., and A. Hastings. 1970. Electromyographic evidence of cerebral malfunction in migraine due to egg allergy. *Medical Annals District Columbia* 39(8):437-41.

Koehler, S., and A. Glaros. 1988. The effect of aspartame on migraine headache. *Headache* 28:10-13.

Kohlenberg, R.J. 1982. Tyramine sensitivity in dietary migraine: a critical review. *Headache* 22:30-4.

Kountz, W.B. 1951. *Thyroid Function and its Possible Role in Vascular Degeneration.* Charles C. Thomas, Springfield, Ill.

Lake-Bakaar, G., et al. 1982. Origin of circulating serum immunoreactive trypsin in man. *Dig. Dis. Sci.* 27(2):143-48.

Langer, S.E., and J.F. Scheer. 1984. *Solved: The Riddle of Illness.* Keats Publishing, Inc., New Canaan, Conn.

Lessof, M.H., Wraith, D.G., Merrett, T.G., et al. 1980. Food allergy and intolerance in 100 patients—local and systemic effects. *Q.J. Med.* 49:259-71.

Lessof, M.H. (ed). 1983. *Clinical Reactions to Foods.* John Wiley & Sons, Chichester.

Lewit, K. 1979. Needle effect in relief of myofascial pain. *Pain* 6:83-90.

Liener, I.E. (ed). 1969. *Toxic Constituents of Plant Foodstuffs.* Academic Press, New York.

Lipton, R., Newman, L., Cohen, J., et al. 1989. Aspartame as a dietary trigger of headache. *Headache* 29:90-2.

Littlewood, J., Glover, V., and M. Sandler. 1982. Platelet phenolsulphotransferase deficiency in dietary migraine. *Lancet* 1:983-86.

Liu, V.J.K., and R.P. Abernathy. 1982. Chromium and insulin in young subjects with normal glucose tolerance. *Am. J. Clin. Nutr.* 35:661-7.

Livingston, J.N., and B.J. Purvis. 1980. Effects of wheat germ agglutinin on insulin binding and insulin sensitivity of fat cells. *Am. J. Physiol.* 238:267-75.

Maher, T., and R. Wurtman. 1987. Possible neurologic effects of aspartame, a widely used food additive. *Envir. H. Per.* 75:53-7.

Makuta, M., et al. 1986. Application of eicosapentaenoic acid to health food. *Jpn. Sudo. Saiensu* 25(1):29-35.

Male, D., and I.M. Roitt. 1979. Analysis of the components of immune complexes. *Mol. Immunol.* 16:197.

Manington, E., Horn, M., and M. Wilkinson, eds. 1970. In: Cochrane, A.L., ed. *Third Migraine Symposium 1969.* Heinemann, London.

Mansfield, J. 1990. *Migraine and the Allergy Connection.* Healing Arts Press, Rochester, Vermont.

Mansfield, L.E., Vaughan, T.R., Waller, S.F., et al. 1985. Food allergy and adult migraine: double-blind and mediator confirmation of an allergic etiology. *Ann. Allergy* 55:126-29.

Mansfield, L.E. 1987. The role of food allergy in migraine: a review. *Ann. Allergy* 58:313-16.

Mansfield, L.E. 1988. Food allergy and headache. *Postgraduate Medicine* 83(7):46-55.

Martinez, O.B., MacDonald, A.C., et al. 1985. Dietary chromium and effect of chromium supplementation on glucose tolerance of elderly Canadian women. *Nutrition Research* 5:609-20.

May, C.D., and S.A. Block. 1978. A modern clinical approach to food hypersensitivity. *Allergy* 33:166.

Medina, J., and S. Diamond. 1978. The role of diet in migraine. *Headache* 18(1):31-4.

Melzack, R. 1981. Myofascial trigger points: relation to acupuncture and mechanism of pain. *Arch. Phys. Med. Rehabil.* May, Vol. 62 (symposium).

Merrett, J., Peatsfield, R.C., Clifford Rose, F., et al. 1983. Food related antibodies in headache patients *J. Neurol. Neurosurg. Psych.* 46:738-42.

Middleton, E. 1984. The flavonoids, trends in pharmaceutical science. *Science* 5:335-8.

Mike, N., Haeney, M.R., Goodwin, B.J.F., et al. 1983. Soya protein antibodies in man: their occurrence and possible relevance in coeliac disease. In: *The Second Fisons Food Allergy Workshop.* Medicine Publishing Foundation, Oxford.

Moffett, A.M., Swash, M., and D.F. Scott. 1974. Effect of chocolate in migraine: a double blind study. *J. Neurol. Neurosurg. Psych.* 37:445-8.

Moncada, S., et al. 1986. Leucocytes and tissue injury: The use of eicosapentaenoic acid in the control of white cell activation. *Wien. Klin. Wochenschr.* 98(4):104-06.

Monro, J., Brostoff, J., Carini, C., et al. 1980. Food allergy in migraine: study of dietary exclusion and RAST. *Lancet* 2:1-4.

Monro, J., Carini, C., and J. Brostoff. 1984. Migraine is a food-allergic disease. *Lancet* 2:719-21.

Monte, W.C. 1984. Aspartame: Methanol and the public health. *J. Appl. Nutr.* 36:42-53.

Morley, J.E. 1982. Food Peptides—a new class hormones? *J.A.M.A.* 17:2379-80.

Nicklas, R.A. 1989. Sulfites: a review with emphasis on biochemistry and clinical application. *Allergy Proc.* 10(5):349-55.

Noah, N.D., et al. 1980. Food poisoning from raw kidney beans. *Br. Med. J.* 2:236-7.

Nylander, M. 1986. Mercury in pituitary glands of dentists. *Lancet* 478:442 Feb.

Oelgoetz, A.W., et al. 1935. The treatment of food allergy and indigestion of pancreatic origin with pancreatic enzymes. *Am. J. Digest. Dis. Nutr.* 2:422-6.

Oelgoetz, A.W., et al. 1936. Further studies in food allergy. *Med. Rec.* 143:20-25.

Oelgoetz, A.W., et al. 1936. Etiology and treatment of food allergy. *Southwestern Med.* 20:463-5.

Oelgoetz, A.W., et al. 1939. Pancreatic enzymes and food allergy. *Med. Rec.* 150:276-9.

Offenbacher, E.G., Rinko, C.J., et al. 1985. The effects of inorganic chromium and brewer's yeast on glucose tolerance, plasma lipids and plasma chromium in elderly subjects. *Am. J. Clin. Nutr.* 42:454-461.

Paganelli, R., Levinsky, R.J., Brostoff, J., et al. 1983. Immune complexes containing food proteins in normal and atopic subjects. *Lancet* 1:1270-72.

Pinckney, E.R. 1983. The accuracy and significance of medical testing. *Arch. Int. Med.* 143(3):512.

Podell, R.N. 1984. Is migraine a manifestation of food allergy? *Postgraduate Med.* 75(4):221-25.

Randolf, T.G., and F. Rawling. 1946. Variations in total leukocytes following test feeding of foods: an appraisal of the individual food test. *Ann. Allergy* 4:163-78.

Randolf, T.G. 1962. *Human Ecology and Susceptibility to the Chemical Environment*. Charles C. Thomas, Springfield, Ill.

Randolf, T.G., Rawling, F., Brostoff, J., et al. 1979. Immune complexes contain food proteins in normal and atopic subjects after oral challenge and effect of sodium cromoglycate on antigen absorption. *Lancet*, pp. 1270-71.

Rapoport, A.M., and F.D. Sheftell. 1990. *Headache Relief*. Simon and Schuster, New York.

Rice, S.L., Eiten Miller, R.R., and P.E. Koehler. 1976. Biologically active amines in food: a review. *J. Milk Food Technol.* 39:353-8.

Rinkel, H.J., Randolf, T.G., and M. Zeller. 1950. *Food Allergy*. Charles C. Thomas, Springfield, Ill.

Rowe, A.H. 1931. *Food Allergy: Its Manifestations, Diagnosis, and Treatment.* Lea & Febiger, Philadelphia.

Rubin, D. 1981. Myofascial trigger point syndromes: an approach to management. *Arch. Phys. Med. Rehabil.* Vol. 62 (symposium) Mar.

Ryan, R.E. 1960. A new approach to the symptomatic treatment of migraine. *Arch. Otolaryng.* 72:325.

Sansum, W.D. 1932. Treatment of indigestion, underweight and allergy with old and new forms of digestive agents. *Southwestern Med.* 16:452-62.

Schwartz, G.R. 1988. *In Bad Taste: The MSG Syndrome.* Signet Books (Penguin Press), New York.

Stevenson, D. 1979. Food allergies and migraine. *Lancet* 14:103.

Stratton, S.A. 1982. Role of endorphins in pain modulation. *J. Ortho. Sports Phys. Ther.* 3(4):200-05.

Swain, A., Dutton, S.P., and A.S. Truswell. 1985. Salicylates in foods. *J. Amer. Diet. Assoc.* 85:950-60.

Taylor, E. 1979. Food additives, allergy and hyperkinesis. *J. Child Psychol. Psychiatry* 20:357-63.

Terano, T., Salmon, J.A., Higgs, G.A., et al. 1986. EPA as a modulator of inflammation: effect upon prostaglandin and leukotriene synthesis. *Biochem. Pharm.* 35(3):779-85.

Todd, L.C. 1933. Food allergy with special reference to migraine. *South. Med. Surg.* pp. 587-92.

Travell, J. 1949. Basis for multiple uses of local block of somatic trigger areas (procaine infiltration and ethylchloride spray). *Mississippi Valley Med. J.* 71:12-21.

Travell, J. 1967. Mechanical headache. *Headache* 7:23-29.

Travell, J. 1981. Identification of myofascial trigger point syndrome; a case of atypical facial neuralgia. *Arch. Phys. Med. Rehabil.* V62 (symposium) Mar.

Unger, L., and A.H. Unger. 1951. A new (sublingual) method for controlling the pain of migraine. *Illinois Med. J.* 99:210.

Unger, A.H. 1952. Migraine is an allergic disease. *J. Allergy* 23:429-40.

Unger, L., and J. Cristol. 1970. Allergic Migraine. *Ann. of Allergy* 28:106-08.

Vahlquist, B. 1955. Migraine in children. *Int. Arch. Allergy Appl. Immunol.* 7:348-55.

Vaughan, W.T. 1927. Allergic Migraine. *J.A.M.A.* 88:1383-86.

Walker, W.A. 1981. *Intestinal Transport of Macromolecules. Physiology of the Gastrointestinal Tract.* L.R. Johnson, ed., Raven Press, New York.

Walker, W.A. 1982. Mechanisms of antigen handling by the gut. *Clinics Immunol. Allergy.* 2(1):15-25.

Walzer, A., et al. 1935. Studies in absorption of undigested proteins in human beings; new technique for quantitatively studying absorption and elimination of antigens: preliminary report. *J. Allergy* 6:532-538.

Walzer, M. 1941. Allergy of the abdominal organs. *J. Lab. Clin. Med.* 26:1867.

Warshaw, L., et al. 1971. Small intestinal permeability to macromolecules. *Lab. Invest.* 25:631-39.

Waters, W.E. 1974. *The Epidemiology of Migraine.* Boehringer Ingleheim, Berkshire.

Webber, T.P. 1973. Diagnosis and medication of headache and shoulder-arm-hand syndrome. *J.A.O.A.* 72:697-710.

Weeks, V.D., and J. Travell. 1957. How to give painless injections. In *Amer. Med. Assoc.: Scientific Exhibits.*

Weiser, M.M., and A.P. Douglas. 1976. An alternative mechanism for gluten toxicity in coeliac disease. *Lancet* 1:567.

Werner, S.C., and S.H. Ingbar, eds. 1965. *The Thyroid.* Harper & Row, New York.

Whybrow, M.B., et al. 1969. Mental changes accompanying thyroid gland dysfunction. *Archives of General Psychiatry* 20:48.

Wide L., Bennich, H., and S.G.O. Johansson. 1967. Diagnosis of allergy by an in-vitro test for allergen antibodies. *Lancet* 2:1105.

Wren, J.C. 1968. Thyroid function and coronary atherosclerosis. *J. Amer. Ger. Soc.* 16:696-704.

Wurtman, R.J., and J.J. Wurtman. 1983. Physiological and Behavioral Effects of Food Constituents. *Nutrition and the Brain.* Vol. 6 Raven Press, New York.

Zioudrou, C., and W.A. Klee. 1979. Possible roles of peptides derived from food proteins in brain function. *Nutrition and the Brain.* 4:125-52.

Index

A

Acidophilus, 12
AC Grace Co., 135
Acupuncture, vii, 52, 85, 86
Addicts, 48
  to wheat, 55
  to drugs, 74
  to sugar, 99
Addisons's Disease, 72
Adrenal cortex, 71
Adrenalin, 71, 106, 107
Adrenal Insufficiency Exam, 77
Adrenal medulla, 71
Adrenal Metabolic Research Society, 72
Adrenals, 9, 10, 62, 70, 71, 72, 73, 74, 75, 76, 79, 102, 104, 107
  cortical insufficiency, 16
Aflatoxin, 9
Alcohol, 20, 32, 33, 47, 48, 49, 74, 77, 101, 112, 123
  beverages, 21, 117
  a solvent, 43
Aldehydes, 43
Alkaloids, 9, 43
Allergens, 26, 69
Allergy, 7, 27, 53, 54, 56, 57, 58, 59, 60, 70, 75, 76, 79, 94, 99, 103
  food, vii, viii, ix, 19, 28, 29, 31, 42, 43, 45, 46, 54, 114
  and chemicals, 6
  to synthetics, 18
  hidden, 21
  to metal, 50
Aluminum, 8, 70
Alzheimer's disease, 37
American Dental Association, 52
American Indians, 14
American Spoon Foods, 134
Amines, 43
Amino acids, 25, 30, 93, 100, 107
  eight essential, 105
  See also specific amino acids
Anaphylactic shock, 34

Anemia, 16, 29, 96, 102
  pernicious, 28
Aneurysms, x, 15
Angiographs, x, 15
Annals of Allergy, 19
Annato, 41
Antibiotics, 27, 28, 101
  toxicity of, 59
Antifreeze, 41
Antigen-antibody complex, 26
Antigens, 25, 31
  food, 29, 32
  protein, 44
Arlington Preventive Medicine Center, 137
Arsenic, 8
Arteries, ix, 20, 21, 25, 31, 44, 45, 67, 88, 91, 109
  supply digestive organs, 30
Arterioles, 22
Arthritis, ix, 75, 82, 83, 88, 107, 112
  rheumatoid, 28, 70
Artificial colorings, 39, 40
Aspirin, ix, 9, 28, 32, 39, 42, 44, 47, 49, 54, 60, 94, 101, 106, 109, 111, 116
  faddism, ix
  epidemic, ix
Asthma, 22, 82
Atherosclerosis, 67, 70

B

Bacteria, 26, 27, 29, 32, 108
  beneficial, 29, 30
Barnes, Dr. Broda, 64, 67
Behavioral disorders, 22
  due to MSG, 37
Bifidus, 29
  See also bacteria
Biofeedback, vii, viii
Bioflavonoids, 45
Biological amines, 9
Biotech, 134
Biotin, 105

Birth control pills (BCP), 21, 28, 112
  users of, 22, 98
Bleach, 49
Blood clots, x, 5, 109, 110
Blood sugar, 2, 6, 7, 10, 61, 71, 76,
  102, 103
  low, 75
  fluctuations in, 76
  regulating mineral, 101
Blood tests, x, 15, 47, 63
  analysis, 16
  specialized, 23
Blood thinners, 109
B-lymphocytes, 26
Brain, x, 5, 8, 10, 20, 31, 45, 50, 51,
  53, 55, 61, 62, 68, 75, 85, 91, 101,
  103, 106, 109, 112
  and membranes, 18, 26
  tissue damage to, 21, 37, 48
  hemorrhage, 44
  function of, 46
Brain infection headaches, 5
Brain scans, x, 6, 15, 54
Brain tumor, x, 5, 6, 15, 115
Brown, Dr., 19
Butter Yellow, 41

C

Cadmium, 8, 70
Calcium, 9, 67, 79, 96, 97, 98, 99,
  105
Cancer, 15, 28, 32, 41, 48, 75,
  112
Carbohydrate intolerance, 16
Carbohydrate metabolism, 67, 73
Carbon dioxide (CO2), 7
Carbon monoxide (CO), 7
Carcinogens, 39, 41
Cardiovascular Research, 103, 135
Casey, Edgar, 82
CAT scans, x, 6, 15, 54
Causes, vii, viii, x, 1, 4, 5, 15, 21,
  23, 45, 54, 75 , 116
  intracranial, 5
  biological, 13
  medical, 14
  of disease, 16
  medical diagnosis of, 17
  of migraine, 20, 48, 50, 75, 115
Celiac/ sprue, 31, 54
  See also gluten intolerance

Central nervous system (CNS), 9, 91,
  106, 109
Cerebral hemorrhage, 15
Charing Cross Hospital, 21
Chemical hepatitis, 33
Chemicals, 7, 9, 20, 21, 35, 39, 42, 45,
  46, 48, 49, 50, 54, 68, 71, 76, 85, 103,
  104, 111, 114, 115
  industrial/ commercial, 8
  agricultural, 8, 32
  allergies to, 18, 23
  ingesting, 25
  noxious agent, 26
  toxic, 31, 36, 41, 112
  synthetic, 40
  of the brain, 69
  neurohormones, 75
Chemical sensitivity, 6, 47
Childhood hyperactivity, 39
Chinese Restaurant Syndrome, 37
Chiropractic, vii
  manipulative treatments, 81, 83, 85,
    86, 87, 91
Cholesterol, 10, 30, 67, 97, 111
Chromium, 97, 101
Cigarette smoke, 9, 77, 112, 117
Circulatory system, 30, 67, 109
Citrus oils, 43
Cluster headaches, 5
Cobalt, 97
Cocaine, 49
Cocoa (Chocolate), 21, 43, 44, 47,
  55, 57, 101, 114, 118, 133
Coffee, 18, 42, 43, 54, 58, 114,
  117, 124, 133
Collagen, 44
  See also protein
Coleman's Organic Beef, 134
College Pharmacy, 138
Colon, 11, 12, 26
Colonic cephalalgia, 11
Colostrum, 29
Constipation, 2, 3, 66, 77, 87,
  88
  headaches due to, 11, 12
Copper, 8, 63, 64, 96, 97
Cortisol, 71, 72
Cortisone, 71, 72
  shots, 90
Cousins, Norman, 17
Crack, 49
Cranial-sacral treatment, 81, 82
Cribiform plate, 7

Cristol, Joel, 19
Cushing's disease, 5, 72

Dura, 86, 87
Dyer, Wayne, 17

D

DDS-acidophilus, 29
DDT, 45, 46
Dental amalgam, 50, 51, 52
Diabetes, 70, 76, 107, 109, 112
Diagnos-Techs, 138
Diarrhea, 3, 38, 77, 100
Digestion, 62
  disorders of, ix
  disturbances of, 2, 3, 6, 16
  problems of, 7
  analysis of, 16
  impaired, 25
Digestive tract, 9
Dioxin, 49, 70
Disease, vii, ix, x, 5, 6, 14, 30, 39, 80,
  107, 114, 117
  organic, 13
  life-threatening, 15
  causation of, 16
  allergic, 19
  due to reduced levels of S-IgA, 28
  of the liver, 32
  neurological, 37, 46
  vascular, 67
  clinical, 68
  due to thyroid failure, 70
  See also specific diseases
Dissecting cervical and/or
  cranial arteries, 44
Diuretics, 9, 101
Doctor's Data, 138
Drugs, x, 18, 31, 36, 44, 48, 49, 95,
  101, 111, 113, 115
  Cafergot, ix, 116
  Inderal, ix, 116
  Midrin, ix, 116
  Valium, ix, 68, 69, 116
  cortisone, 9, 32, 45
  Indocin, 9, 32, 42
  Cardiazem, 9
  Coumadin, 9
  Hydralazine, 9
  recreational or medical, 32
  heavy dosages of, 33
  dependencies, 47
  radioactive iodine, 64
  Xanax, 68, 69, 116

E

Eat Right or Die Young, 79, 102
Ecological Formulas, 100, 108, 135
Eczema, 22, 107
EEG, 15
Egger, J. Dr., 22
Electrical currents, 51, 52
Electromyograph (EMG) 45, 46
ELISA test, 23, 24
Encephalitis, 2
Endocrine glands, 61, 70
Endocrinology, 61
Endorphins, 68, 106
Enkephalins, 106
Environmental Dental Association
  (EDA), 53
Enzymatic Therapies, 108, 135
Enzymes, 25, 30, 70, 93, 106, 107, 108
  system for detoxifying, 35
  pancreatic, 50
Eosinophillic Myalgic Syndrome (EMS),
  105
Ergotamine, 9
Esophagus, 26
Estrogens, 63, 98
Extremities, 2, 3

F

Fallopian tubes, 44
Fast food, 37, 41, 42, 58, 59
  chains, 48
Fasting, 23, 24
Fats, 31, 73, 94, 109, 110, 112
Fatty acids, 30, 93
  essential, 64, 103, 112
Feingold, Dr., 39
Fever, 69
Feverfew, 94
Fiber, 12
Fish oils (EPA/DHA), 109, 110, 111
Flavonoids, 43, 95
Folic acid, 28, 44, 45, 63, 64, 105
Food, 46, 49, 100, 108, 109, 114, 124,
  125, 126
  allergies, vii, viii, 16, 22, 23, 43, 57,
  59, 115, 117

reactions, vii, 77
extracts, 14, 24
additives, 20, 33, 34, 35, 40, 41, 42
which causes migraine, 21
allergenic, 22
ingesting, 25
noxious agent, 26
colorings, 41
sensitivity, 47
for the brain, 103
list of- to evaluate allergies, 128
Food allergy testing, 15, 59
Food Intolerance Test, 23, 24, 54, 128
Food and Drug Administration (FDA),
50, 105
Food dyes, 20, 39, 41, 42, 43, 47
See also artificial colorings
Formaldehyde, 7
Frontal headaches, 6
Fumes, 7, 8, 18, 42, 114
Fungus, 43

G

Gamma linolenic acid
(GLA), 112
Garlic, 79, 95
Ginger, 11, 94, 95, 132
Glucose, 10, 44, 75, 101, 103
Gluten, 44
grains that contain, 31
Gluten intolerance, 31, 54
See also celiac/sprue
Gold fillings, 50, 52
Goltman, 18
Grant, Dr. Ellen, 21, 22
Gut bombs, 37, 74

H

Hair analysis, 9, 15,
toxic metal analysis, 16
Harrison's Textbook of Internal Medi-
cine, 6, 62
Heart disease, 2, 67, 74, 75, 109
Heavy metals, 8, 70
See also specific heavy metals
Hemoglobin, 7
Henry's Farms, 134
Herbs, 14, 93, 94, 95
See also specific herbs
Heroin, 49

High blood pressure, 2, 5, 21, 70
hypertension, 16
Histamine, 20, 104
History, 14, 15
Homeopathy, vii
Honey, 76, 132
Hormones, 53, 61, 70, 71, 76, 106
disorders of, 6
disturbances of, 7
adrenal and thyroid, 10, 67, 69, 70,
73, 75, 103, 104
glandular function of, 16, 62
dysfunction of, 16
sex, 63
cortical, 72
secretion of, 107
Hospital for Sick Children and Institute
of Child Health, 22
Hydrogenated oils, 42, 112
Hyperthyroidism, 63, 69
Hypertrophy, 62
Hypoadrenocorticism, 72, 75
Hypochondriac, 6, 19
Hypoglycemia, 5, 70, 75, 76, 101, 107
Hypothalamus, 61, 62
Hypothyroidism, 5, 16, 63, 64, 65, 67,
68, 70, 88, 115
Hypothyroid Questionnaire, 65, 66
Hypotension, 16

I

Igram, Dr. Cass, 79, 102, 137
Immune complexes, 26, 30
Immune system, x, 9, 26, 34, 47, 69,
71, 72, 79, 108
diseases of, 53
Immunoglobulins, 26, 27, 28, 29
Infections, 5, 6, 31, 32, 114, 115
viral, x, 2, 46
Injury
due to car accident, 1
Insulin, 10, 44
Intestinal villi, 31
Intestines, ix, 11, 29, 33, 41, 44, 56,
57, 72
malabsorption in, 16
digestive juices in, 25
small, 26, 31
human, 27, 29, 43
overgrowth in, 30
Iodine, 64
Iron, 96, 97, 102

J

Joseph, Dr. Beverly, 137
Journal of the American Medical Association, 19
Junk food, 48, 58, 59, 73, 112
Juvenile diabetes, 48

K

Kidneys, x, 26, 51, 71, 72, 103, 106
  damage to, 52, 53
Klaire Labs, 108, 135
Kuppfer cells, 32
Kyodophilus, 29
Kyolic-EPA, 111
Kyolic garlic, 111

L

Lactobacillus acidophilus, 29
  See also bacteria
Land O' Lakes, 41
LaRoche, Dr., 19
Lead, 8, 70
Learning disorders, 39, 48
Lemon, 43, 44, 54, 130
  allergy to, 53, 57
Licorice root, 11, 79, 95
Limes, 43, 57, 130
Liver, ix, 9, 10, 11, 26, 27, 33, 34, 44,
  51, 62, 69, 72, 95
  alteration in, 22
  a formidable foe, 32
Lou Gehrig's disease, 37
Lower back, 1
  strain/sprain, 86
Lumbar puncture
  (spinal tap), 2
Lungs, 7, 34, 41
  disease of, 109
Lymphatic vessels, 31
Lymph nodes, 26, 27, 69

M

Magnesium, 9, 79, 94, 96, 97, 98, 100,
  101, 103
Magnesium Taurate, 100

Manganese, 96, 97
Mansfield, Dr., 20, 21, 117
Massage, viii
Master of Metabolism, 70
  See also thyroid
Maulfair, Jr., Dr. Conrad G., 137
Medication, viii, 2, 33, 60, 64, 79, 82,
  85, 92, 94
  which reduce S-IgA levels, 28
  potentially toxic, 45
  anti-depressants/anti-anxiety, 68
Meningitis, x, 15
Menner Chiropractic, 137
Mercury, 8, 51, 52, 53, 70
Methanol, 50
  See also wood alcohol
Microbes, 26, 27, 32, 69, 108
  noxious, 30
Migraine headaches, vii,viii, ix, x, 1, 2,
  3, 4, 14, 15, 16, 25, 28, 32, 38, 42, 55,
  56, 58, 60, 67,70, 72, 75, 89, 93, 107,
  110, 114, 117
  causation of, 18
  due to food allergy, 18, 19, 23, 43, 44,
    101, 102, 104
  chronic, 20, 45
  due to BCP, 21
  childhood, 22, 46, 47
  due to S-IgA deficiency, 27
  resistant to, 29
  due to gluten intolerance, 31
  treatment of, 32
  alcohol precipitates, 32
  due to hormones, 61
  due to hypothyroidism, 63, 65
  due to hypoglycemia, 76
  magnesium for, 100
Migraine Intensity Exam, 2
Migraine personality, 19, 20
Migraine provokers
  (list of), 43
Migraineurs, vii, 16, 17, 19, 23, 42, 61,
  95
Miller, Dr. Norman, 137
Mineral Deficiency Exam, 96
Minerals, 9, 30, 31, 34, 79, 93, 95, 96,
  100, 101, 102, 105
  assessment for, 15
  trace, 35
  megadoses of, 52
  anti-migraine, 94, 97
  See also individual minerals
Mold residues, 43

Molybdenum, 35, 97
Monro, Dr., 21
Montefiore Medical Headache Unit, 21
Mother's milk, 29
Mouth, 26
MRI, x, 54
MSG, 20, 36, 37, 38, 40, 42, 43, 47, 58, 125

N

Narcotics, 68, 116
  Demerol, ix, 68
Natural flavors, 37, 38
Nature's Way, 135
Nausea, 1, 3, 15, 38, 57, 58
Neck, 11, 31, 38, 44, 78, 82, 83, 86, 87, 88, 91, 106
  stiff, 15
  injuries to, 84
  artery surgery, 85
Nerves, 36, 50, 51, 85, 88, 96, 97, 100, 117
  brain and spinal, 8
  impulses of, 9
  peripheral, 10
  vagus, cranial, colonic, 11
  irritation, 44
  function of, 46
  irritants to, 55
  conduction, 62
  cervical, 84
  tonic for, 94
Nervous system, 45, 48, 52, 71, 97, 98, 100, 106, 109
Ness, 108
Neural Therapy, 89
Neuroactive peptides, 44, 54
Neurotoxin, 36, 51
Neurotransmitter Depletion Syndrome, 68
Neurotransmitters, 68, 103, 106
  levels of, 107
Niacin, 64, 105
Nickel, 8, 50, 52
Nitrates, 9, 124
Nitrites, 20, 42
Noradrenalin, 71, 106
Nutra Sweet, 21, 25, 42, 47, 50
Nutrition, vii
  deficiencies of, 16, 44
  therapy with, 28, 57

Nutritional garbage, 48
Nutitional Testing Laboratories, 138

O

Obesity, 48, 70
Oelgoetz, Dr., 108
Oregon Apiaries
Osteopathic manipulative treatments (OMT), 52, 55, 60, 81, 82, 83, 84, 85, 86, 87, 91
Osteopathy, vii
Ovaries, 44, 62
Oven Poppers, 134
Oxidation, 35
Oxygen (O), 7, 44, 85, 104

P

Pancreas, 10, 11, 25, 50, 62, 72, 108
Pantothene, 103
Pantothenic acid, 28, 79, 90, 102, 103
Parasites, x, 26, 29, 108
  intestinal, 16, 70
Parkinsonism, 37, 107
Pathogens, 27
Peripheral vision, 45, 59
Phenlyalanine (DLPA), 105, 106, 107
Phenylketonuria, 106
Physical examination, 14, 15
Physical therapy, viii
Pituitary gland, 53, 61, 62
Platelets, 20, 21, 24, 75, 103, 110, 111
Polance, Dr. Hal, 89
Potassium, 9, 71, 94, 96, 97
Precipitin, 30
Premenstrual headache, 5
Premenstrual Syndrome (PMS), 2, 61, 63, 66, 78, 105, 112, 115
Prime-Life, 29
Procaine, 90
Prodroma, 1
Proteins, 25, 26, 31, 44, 71, 73, 104, 105, 107, 108
  noxious agent, 26
  S-IgA made from, 28
  from undigested milk, 30
  gluten, 3
  part of food, 43
Psychoanalysis, viii
Pylorospasm, 57

Pylorus, 57
Pyridoxal-5-phosphate
(P-5-P), 103, 104

R

Randolph, Dr. Theron, 19, 23
RAST testing, 23, 24
Rice bran, 102
Ritalin, 39
Red blood cell, 7, 24
Reye's Syndrome, ix, x
Rotation diet, 23
Rowe, 21

S

Saccharin, 25, 50, 58
Salicylate, 20, 39, 47, 59, 126
Schwartz, Dr. George, 36
Scratch testing, 23, 24
Secretory IgA (S-IgA), 26, 28, 30, 31
   immune protein, 27
   good bacteria enhance
   production of, 29
   deficiency of, 57
Selenium, 63, 64, 96, 97
Selye, Hans, 72, 75
Sella tursica, 62
Serotonin, 20, 21
Shaw, George Bernard, 116
Siegel, Bernie, 17
Silicon, 96, 97
Silver-mercury fillings, 50, 52, 53
   See also dental amalgam
Smog headache, 7
Sodium, 71, 97
Spasms, 11
Spinal cord, 10, 11, 45, 84, 85, 86, 91
   lesions of, 83
Spinal manipulation, 82
Spleen, 26, 27, 69, 72
Standard American diet, 63
Still, Andrew Taylor, 13, 80
Stress, viii, 6, 9, 10, 14, 15, 25, 53, 58,
   61,70, 72, 74, 76, 78, 98, 101, 102,
   103, 107, 117
   emotional, 19, 62
   mental, 75
Stomach, ix, 10, 11, 26, 32, 44, 57, 71, 95
   sleeping on, 2
   pain in, 22
   empty, 24

digestive juices in, 25
   cramps in, 38
Stool analysis, 16
Stroke, 15, 109, 110
Structural defects, 6, 7
Structural therapies, 16
Sub-clinical Addison's Disease, 72
Sugars, 30, 36, 42, 47, 49, 57, 58, 59,
   73, 74, 76, 79, 94, 100, 101, 125, 132
   liver synthesizes, 10
   non-protein substance, 25
   white, 27, 96
   high in, 48
   addicts to, 70
Sulfites, 33, 34, 35, 36, 40, 42, 43, 56,
   59, 124
Sulfur, 97
Sulfur dioxide (SO2), 34
Sympathetic fibers, 85
Symptoms, x, 1, 2, 10, 11, 13, 15, 24,
   42, 45, 55, 63, 100, 115
   due to food, 21, 79
   allergy, 23
   due to sulfites, 34
   due to MSG, 37, 38
   due to DDT, 46
   due to mercury intoxication, 53
   due to hypothyroidism, 68
   due to mineral deficiency, 96
   mental, 103
Synthroid, 63

T

Tailbone, 84
   coccyx, 87
Tartrazine, 39
   See also Yellow Dye #5
Taurine, 100
Tea, 18, 42, 127, 133
Tension headaches, 5, 11, 89
Testes, 62
Tests, x, 4, 6, 14, 54, 57
   to rule out serious causes, 15
   to diagnose, 16
   neurological, 45
   for allergies, 55
   of thyroid, 64
The Lancet, 21, 53
The Leaky Gut Syndrome, 29, 32
   leaky gut, 30
Theobromines, 20, 44
Thiamine, 28, 63, 64, 79, 104

Thymus, 10, 62, 69, 72
Thyroid, 9, 62, 63, 64, 67, 69, 70
  thyroiditis of, 16
  disorders of, 65
  function of, 68
Thyroxin, 69, 106
Tin, 50, 52
Tintera, John M.D., 72, 75
TMJ Syndrome, 87, 89
Tobacco, 43, 54, 59, 133
  leaf of, 9
Toxins, 32, 42, 52, 69, 114
  of nerve, 37, 50
Traumatic headaches, 5
Treatment, 1, 79, 113, 117
  alternative, vii
Trigger point, 88, 89, 90
  injections, 52, 55, 86, 87, 92
  therapy, 60, 83, 85, 91
Triglyceride levels, 67, 97
Tryptophan, 105
Turmeric, 94, 95
Tylenol, ix, 9, 42, 60, 106, 116
Tyramines, 20, 33
Tyrosine, 105, 106, 107

U

Underarm temperature test, 64
Unger, Leon, 19, 20
University of Tennessee, 100
Urine tests, x, 15
  analysis, 16
U.S. Bison Company, 134
Uterus, 22, 26, 30, 44

V

Vagal cephalalgia, 11
Vaughn, Dr., 20
Veins, x, 21, 45, 88, 91
  uterine, 22
Vertebra, 84, 85, 86
Vitaline, 108
Viruses, 26, 108
Visual disturbances, 1, 3, 15, 57, 58, 59
Vitamins, 28, 30, 31, 82, 93, 102, 123
  assessment for, 15
  B (complex), 45, 103
  megadoses of, 52
  See also specific vitamins
Vitamin A, 9, 28, 45, 63, 64, 79
Vitamin B-2, 63, 64, 105

Vitamin B-6, 28, 63, 64, 79, 102, 103, 104
  deficiency, 112
Vitamin B-12, 28, 34, 35, 64, 90
Vitamin C, 28, 44, 45, 64, 79, 102, 104
Vitamin D, 98
Vitamin E, 28, 45, 64, 79, 102, 104, 110, 111
Vitamin K, 45
Vomiting, 1, 3, 15, 57

W

Wakunaga Corporation, 29, 135
Water, 12, 35, 71, 82, 96, 100, 103
  chlorine in, 27, 112
  spring, 38
  and sugar, 73
  sterile salt, 90
Watercress, 99, 131
Whiplash, 1, 83
  acceleration-deceleration injury, 84
White blood cells, 24, 26, 69, 104, 108
  landlocked, 32
  synthesis of, 71
Wine, 9, 33, 35, 42, 43, 48, 114, 120, 123, 127
  coolers, 40
Withdrawal, 48
Wolfe, Dr. Harold, 91
Wood alcohol, 50
  See also methanol

X

X-rays, 15, 62

Y

Yeasts, x, 26, 29, 43, 58, 108, 122, 123
  Candida albicans, 27, 28, 59, 70, 89
  overgrowth of, 28
  baker's, 55, 132
  chronic infection, 56, 112
  brewer's, 102, 132
Yellow Dye #5, 39, 40
  See also tartrazine

Z

Zinc, 50, 63, 96, 97, 112